FIVE THOUSAND
YEARS
OF MEDICINE

FIVE THOUSAND
YEARS
OF MEDICINE

by Gerhard Venzmer

TRANSLATED BY MARION KOENIG

MACDONALD · LONDON

Made and printed in Great Britain by
Tonbridge Printers Ltd
Peach Hall Works, Tonbridge, Kent

Contents

Rhazi and Avicenna. The medical school of Salerno was the seed from which the medical faculties of the future were to spring the despised guild of barbers to that of medical surgeons. The Frenchman, Ambroise Paré, the 'father of surgery', completes this task and creates an entirely modern sounding 'comprehensive treatment'

Boerhaave, who turned his academy in Leiden into 'the cradle of our modern clinic'. Albrecht Haller of Switzerland, the first man in medical history to write a systematic manual of physiology

9

Anatomy through his 'theory of membranes'. Corvisart, Napoleon's personal physician, amplifies Auenbrugger's physical method of diagnostics Laennec invents the stethoscope directs German anatomical, physiological and medical research into a truer scientific attitude. Johann Lukas Schönlein also decides the direction which the development of natural science in German medical research is to take. First signs of the era of bacteriology

Research into vitamins and hormones directs doctors' attention back to the totality of the patient

I

*The art of healing was practised even in
prehistoric times. The witch-doctor in
the cave of Les Trois Frères.*

On 20 July 1914, Comte Henri
de Bégouen, professor of ancient history at the University of
Toulouse, and his three sons, were on a trip through the valley
of the Ariège, a tributary of the Garonne in the Pyrennean foothills south of the town. The day was hot and they sat down to
rest not far from Montesquieu-Avantès. While they were sitting
by the roadside, a farmer came by. He told them there was no
need for them to sit there in the heat. Not far away was a much
more comfortable resting place – where cool air came up out of
the ground on even the hottest day.

Professor Bégouen pricked up his ears. Cool air blowing up
out of the ground surely could only come from a cave... A
few moments later they came upon the *trou souffleur*. The stones,
half-concealing the opening, were cleared away and Professor
Bégouen was proved right: a large crack led down into the earth.
The archaeologist's interest was aroused; ropes and a lantern were
obtained. One of his sons was carefully lowered down the fissure
with a rope secured round him. He went down about sixty feet
before reaching the bottom; then he untied the rope and began
to explore. In suspense, and with some anxiety, those who had
stayed behind waited for a signal. It was more than an hour,
however, before there was a movement on the rope. The boy in

the cave retied it round himself and was pulled up into the day-
light by the others. On arriving at the top, he was at first too
excited to speak. 'The walls are covered with pictures, hundreds
of them,' he finally blurted out. Time was to show that he was
not exaggerating.

Among the countless paintings on the walls of the cave – which,
because of the manner of its discovery, was later named *Les Trois
Frères* – there is a picture which may well be the oldest known
representation of a medicine man: an Ice-Age witch-doctor wear-
ing an animal mask. The mask, with its big, round eyes and
pointed beard, is in the form of a bison's face surmounted with
bison's horns. The bison's hump is clearly recognizable. A bison's
tail swings down, the front legs end in a bison's cloven hooves.
But the posture of this bison-man is human, erect. The feet, also,
are human.

The discovery of this Ice-Age doctor who lived and worked
more than seventeen thousand years ago, confirms, yet again,
that sickness already existed in those early days of man's development. It makes nonsense of the theory, often put forward, that,
when man was still living in a state of nature, there was no such
thing as illness, and that it only came later with civilization.
Scientists, it is true, did not need to discover a medicine man
in the cave of *Les Trois Frères* in order to appreciate for how
long ill health has existed. A vast body of evidence is there to
prove that illnesses are even older than human beings, that they
are almost as old as life itself. As palaeontologists bring more
long-forgotten worlds to light, it becomes still clearer that hundreds of millions of years ago the same illnesses existed as those
which the doctor encounters in his consulting-room today.

Even the bacteria which cause so many infectious diseases have
existed from time immemorial: they have been found fossilized
in Cambrian rock layers. These layers are estimated to be five
hundred million years old. There is still some doubt, of course,
whether the fission-fungi of those times were already active in

causing sickness or whether they were harmless to other living organisms.

In Devonian and Silurian fossil shells, estimated to be three hundred and fifty million years old, we even discover ravages apparently caused by parasites. The immense length of time during which disease has existed is shown still more clearly by relics dating back to the beginning of the Cretaceous period, that is to say about one hundred and fifty million years ago. These are the remains of the legendary saurians, reminiscent of our present-day ideas of dragons, who lived in the tropical climate of those times. A whole catalogue of ailments can be identified on the remains of these grotesque giants of up to 115 feet in length, whose fossil skeletons can be seen in our museums.

For obvious reasons, the ailments identified on these saurian relics are chiefly bone complaints: there are signs that inflammation of the bone and bone tumours were not infrequent. The remains of a dinosaur's tail, discovered in Wyoming, U.S.A., were found to contain bone tumours which had made it so rigid that the creature had clearly been unable to move, and so had met its death. Even caries were found, a form of decay which we nowadays regard as exclusively due to civilization.

When the Mesozoic era came to an end, the age of the saurians was over. The Tertiary era saw the domination of the mammals whose fossil remains, too, show traces of several illnesses; again, chiefly diseases of the bone, particularly inflammations and tumours. Arthritic deformities are especially numerous in the remains of cave bears dating back to the Diluvial epoch.

Directly the first human beings appear, at the end of the Tertiary era and the beginning of the Quaternary Ice Age, roughly half a million years ago, there is evidence of more diseases. The skeletal remains of Pithecanthropus, which the Dutch doctor and palaeontologist Dubois excavated in Java during the 1890s had, on its thigh-bone, a swelling that could only be diagnosed as a tumour.

If any further proof is needed that arthritis, which is so prevalent today, was a primeval illness, this is produced by another race of early man. Traces of Neanderthal man were first found during the middle of the last century by a German secondary-school teacher, Fuhlrott, in caves discovered in the Neander valley at Mettman, between Düsseldorf and Elberfeld. Later, more were found on sites in Thuringia, Belgium, the South of France, Italy, Spain, Czechoslovakia, the Balkans, the Middle East, North and Central Africa and, again, in Java. Many of these skeletal remains proved without doubt that Neanderthal man was often afflicted with arthritis.

During the last centuries of the Ice Age and the first of the Old Stone Age, Neanderthal man was replaced by a new race, the direct ancestor of homo sapiens. And, judging by his remains, he too was plagued by a multitude of bone diseases such as arthritis, tumours, spinal tuberculosis, sinusitis, congenital dislocation of the hip-joint, osteomyelitis, and deformities such as cleft spine. Rickets probably also existed. The rich haul of relics dating from that period, and excavated from caves, conveys to us a vivid picture of the lives and thoughts of those Stone-Age men. In them the artistic spirit stirred for the first time, inspiring them to record in pictures and carvings what they had experienced and observed. These people, in whom at one stroke a sense of art was born, and who knew how to form works of art after practically no period of transition, how to use fire and make remarkable tools and implements out of bone and flint, have, in addition, left us the first traces of a healing activity through the witch-doctor in the entrance to *Les Trois Frères* cave.

We do not know how the Stone-Age medicine men treated their patients. It is quite possible that they already knew about the healing properties of certain herbs, that with such remarkably fine flint instruments as their stone knives they undertook simple operations such as the lancing of abscesses and so on, and perhaps even sewed up wounds with bone needles. There is also evidence dating back to those times of well-healed fractures which would seem to indicate experience in setting at rest or in splints.

Most astonishing of all, however, is the thought that the healers of the New Stone Age ventured to perform an operation which even today counts among the most difficult and risky of all surgical interventions: that of trepanning, or boring a hole into the skull. A surprisingly large number of prehistoric skulls with bored holes have been found in New Stone Age excavations in France, Spain, Germany, Austria, Russia and Poland; occasional examples have also come to light in England and Peru. Probably these early doctors tackled such an operation by boring a series of small holes in a circle so that they eventually met and made it possible for a circular disc of bone to be lifted out. After its removal, this disc was often given an additional hole and worn round the neck as an amulet.

One can imagine the dreadful pain which the unanaesthetized patient had to endure during these operations. In the past, nobody could understand how a trepanning operation with such instruments was even possible. But more recent reviews of the procedure have shown that in fact a properly worked flint could bore a hole through a human skull in five to six minutes. Many people must undoubtedly never have survived trepanation, but the quite considerable number of skulls with well-healed bore holes are sufficient evidence that the patient also frequently survived this critical operation.

Archaeologists are by no means in agreement in their theories as to why such an excessively painful and dangerous operation was undertaken relatively often. A likely explanation, for example, might be that after skull injuries, splinters of bone were exerting pressure on certain parts of the brain and so causing convulsions. Or perhaps the prehistoric medicine men may have assumed, when confronted by patients suffering from fits of madness, epilepsy or unbearable headaches such as migraines, that an evil spirit had made its home inside the skull and a hole would offer it a way of escape. Finally, there is a body of opinion which believes that trepanning was only performed for ritual purposes. All points of view, however, can be reduced to one common denominator: the realization that in its beginnings, the art of healing was imbued with an aura of magic and lay in the hands of the priests. No evidence of limb amputation can be found in Stone-Age bones, although experiments made in recent years have proved that it is possible to saw through the bones of the upper arm with a suitably prepared flint. In some caves, however, singular paintings of finger amputations have been found. But medical opinion inclines to the view that such amputations were undertaken not for medical but again only for ritual purposes. In this connection it is of no small interest that even today some tribes of Papuans, living in New Guinea, who still lead entirely Stone-Age lives, practise finger amputation as a mark of mourning or sorrow.

The development of a system of medical thought depends on a body of transmitted knowledge to which further additions can be made. This, however, presupposes a record; that is to say, the existence of writing. The oldest known scripts appear on clay tablets and clay fragments which were found in Abraham's town, the Chaldean town of Ur in Mesopotamia, during excavations made after the First World War. In general it seems that the cradle of civilization lay in the Tigris and Euphrates valleys, well before the dawn of Egyptian culture; the development of the Sumerian culture began in the fourth millennium BC. Royal tombs dating from about 3500 BC have revealed funeral gifts of unbelievable artistic worth and technical perfection, made by goldsmiths of considerable ability and portraying men and animals in forms which could only have been created by people belonging to a sophisticated culture. We must thank the Ancient Sumerians' passion for recording all important events in pictures or cuneiform script on clay tablets for our knowledge of the oldest medical activities built on tradition.

2

*The cradle of human civilization and of
the art of healing lay in the river valleys of
Mesopotamia. Medical science created
from knowledge which had been handed
down. Religion, magic and medicine
closely interwoven.*

The history of the Mesopot-
amian river-lands is one of constant change. The Sumerians, who
called themselves 'the black-headed people', migrated to the delta-
lands of the Tigris and Euphrates – nobody knows from where
– and they brought with them considerable artistic gifts. They
knew how to construct a vault, wrote a cuneiform script, were
the originators of the oldest known system of astronomy and
collection of laws, and they created their own literature. When
they arrived, they absorbed the civilization of the Akkadians
who had been living there since the New Stone Age. These
Akkadians were primitive hunter-farmers who still used flint tools,
harvesting their corn with sickles made from flakes of
flint.

The first flowering of the purely Sumerian culture which
followed survived until the middle of the third millennium BC,
when a conqueror came from Format – Sargon or Sharrukin of
Akkad by name – who succeeded in subjugating the Sumerians
and founded a new dynasty. This dynasty remained in power
for two centuries until an invasion of hill people brought it to an

end. When the Akkadian kingdom was destroyed, Sumer experienced a second flowering; then, at the turn of the second millennium BC, it began to fade again. On each occasion, however, the conquerors absorbed a considerable part of the Sumerian civilization. First came the Assyrians and then the Babylonians. Their empire was not overthrown until the sixth century BC, by the Persian king Cyrus, the same king who had conquered Asia Minor. It is possible, therefore, without generalizing, to speak of a Mesopotamian culture, a culture of such richness that its influence extended for more than four thousand years and continues to this day.

Excavations prove, beyond all doubt, that there were doctors in this river valley civilization of 2000 BC. During the second half of the eighteenth century, countless clay tablets bearing cuneiform inscriptions were found in the ruins of the city of Nippur (now called Nuffar). One of these tablets appeared to refer to medical texts. The clay tablet in question remained in the British Museum for decades, but no one succeeded in deciphering the text. A provisional interpretation was undertaken by the English scholar of cuneiform scripts, R. Campbell Thompson, but it was not satisfactory. It was not until 1953 that another expert in cuneiform script, Professor Samuel Noah Kramer of Pennsylvania University, and his colleagues succeeded in unravelling the secret of the mysterious clay tablet. What emerged was sensational for the history of medicine, for it appeared that during the third millennium BC, a regular manual of healing – evidently the oldest in the world – had been engraved on this tablet. The most important part of this medical text was a collection of prescriptions, together with a list of drugs and chemical substances which, in those days thousands of years ago, were used for medical purposes. All in all, the doctors of Ancient Mesopotamia recognized hundreds of medicinal plants of which many are still in use today as, for example, opium poppy, mandragora, henbane, linseed, licorice roots, myrrh, thyme, cassia, colocynth, asafoetida, Indian hemp and belladonna. These vegetable medicines were augmented by such minerals as alum, sulphur, saltpetre and copper.

The existence of an indigenous medical profession in Meso-potamia is also proved by the discovery of medical roll-seals containing descriptions of healing divinities and medical instru-ments, which were found in the innumerable mounds of potsherds excavated in Mesopotamia. Such roll-seals were constantly worn by the ancient inhabitants of the river delta on a cord wound round the wrist. The first list of medical fees known to us is contained in the Codex of Laws of King Hammurabi of Babylon who is said by some archaeologists to have reigned in about 2200 BC, but according to others not until two hundred, three hundred or even five hundred years later. The codex, which evidently incorporated most of the Ancient Sumerian body of ideas, then more than a thousand years old, is chiselled in a cuneiform script approximately seven-and-a-half feet high, into a block of diorite. This block had already been excavated in Susa (now called Shush) at the beginning of the nineteenth century. It had been dragged there by Elamitic conquerors; today it is in Paris, in the Louvre.

Apart from the criminal and civil laws – the laws regarding official duties, marriage and divorce, jurisdiction, farming, trade and shipping – it contains the oldest tariff of charges to survive, amongst which can be found fixed fees for various services, including nine paragraphs devoted to medical fees. These do not merely deal with the fee which the medical practitioner received for work of one kind or another; they also lay down the penalties for the doctor's mistakes, and expressly take into account whether the doctor had been treating a man from the upper classes or a slave. 'If a doctor has treated a man with a metal knife for a severe wound, and has cured the man, or has opened a man's tumour with a metal knife and cured a man's eye; then he shall receive ten shekels of silver.' However, if he performed the same operation on the son of a plebeian, the doctor was paid five shekels and if on a slave only two shekels. 'If a doctor has treated a man with a metal knife for a severe wound, and has caused the man to die, or has opened a man's tumour with a metal knife and destroyed the man's eye; his hands shall be cut off.' The doctor was awarded the same punishment if, as a result of an operation, the patient lost his eyesight. 'If a doctor has treated the slave of a plebeian with a metal knife for a severe wound, and caused him to die; he shall render slave for slave. If he has opened his tumour with a metal knife, and destroyed his eye, he shall pay half his price in silver.' The treatment of broken limbs or intestinal complaints cost five shekels for a master, three shekels for a plebeian and two shekels for a slave. 'If a doctor sees that his patient cannot be cured he must not concern himself with that patient, for the patient will die ... If a man has given his child to a nurse, and the child dies in the hand of the nurse, and the nurse without the knowledge of his father and his mother suckles another child; she shall be prosecuted, and because she has suckled another child without the knowledge of his father and his mother, her breasts shall be cut off.'

Whereas the clay tablet mentioned earlier, dating from 2200 BC and containing a medical text, makes no mention at all of devil worship of black magic, the art of healing as practised in Mesopotamia, like all other early civilizations, was based on a close mixture of religious worship, magic, fear of demons and witchcraft. So it seems that the liberation of medicine from a belief in gods, magic or demons was only to have been a passing phase; and as the healing methods were in the hands of doctor-priests, medical treatment was permeated with magic and ritual.

This phenomenon may seem surprising in such a highly civi-lized people, but will be easier to understand if the beliefs which then prevailed about the nature of disease are taken into account. The whole world was believed to be filled with mysterious forces which controlled everything that happened to men, animals, plants and minerals. A whole host of gods and goddesses could decide about sickness or health, each disease being the province of a different demon. Sometimes the disease was brought by a demon, at other times the disease was itself a demon. The exorcism of evil spirits, disease-bearing demons and devils of all kinds, was the function of the priests – hence the close intermingling of religion, magic and medicine in the minds of all ancient peoples. Obviously a transformation in this respect could only take place after the prevailing outlook on the origin and nature of disease had undergone a radical change.

The magic of numbers was also enjoying a vogue at that time. It is interesting to observe that belief in the unlucky properties of number seven already existed in the Ancient Mesopotamian civilization. On the seventh day of the month the king did not drive out in state in his splendid carriage, nor did he grant audiences on that day. Beliefs surrounding the number seven were later to play an important part in the Hippocratic theory of crises. 'Evil seven' became 'holy seven' and the strange significance of the number seven survives to this day; for seven is the number of days in the week, the number of the Jewish sabbatical year, the number of sacraments in the Roman Catholic Church, the virtues and the deadly sins, etc.

Proof that a belief in the magical properties of the number seven really does go back to the Mesopotamian civilization thousands of years ago, is provided by the old Babylonian invocation for the exorcism of demons, as described by R. Campbell Thompson in his book on the devils of Ancient Babylon. The following magic formula refers to Ea, the divine magician of diseases who, like Aesculapius later in Greece, was claimed by Mesopotamian doctors as their ancestor:

> Seven are they: Seven are they!
> In the Ocean Deep seven are they!
> Battening in Heaven seven are they,
> Bred in the depths of Ocean.
> Nor male nor female are they,
> But are as the roaming windblast,
> No wife have they, no son can they beget;
> Knowing neither mercy nor pity,
> They hearken not to prayer or supplication.

They are as horses reared among the hills . . .
The Evil ones of Ea.
Throne-bearers to the gods are they;
They stand in the highway to befoul the path,
Marching before the Plague God, the mighty warrior of Bel.
Evil are they, evil are they!
Seven are they! Seven are they!
Twice seven are they!

An immense number of such magic formulae have come down to us; there was a different invocation for every occasion, and every convalescent owned a set of rags for the special purpose of misleading the demons. For thousands of evil spirits were always waiting to inject human beings and animals with diseases, to bewitch them, cause mischief and bring about miscarriages, to bring plague and famine to the land.

Divination played an important role in conjecturing the outcome of illnesses and other afflictions. The strangest practices – also encountered among doctors of other civilizations – were employed to this end. Divinations were made from the intestines of sacrificial animals; priests could even distinguish the features of an evil spirit on pieces of gut. The appearance of the liver was also very significant, the study of this organ having been developed into a system which was worked out to the smallest detail. The Ancient Babylonians believed the liver to be the dwelling-place of life and soul; the liver of a sacrificial ram or goat was identified with that of the patient, that is to say, whatever was found in the liver of the creature which had been sacrificed was deemed valid for the patient's liver also. Diagnosis or prognosis was always made from the whole organ and not from an opened or dissected one. Any possible deviation from the normal shape or form was carefully observed, as were the lines which limit the individual lobes of the liver, the way in which they branch, and any other such anomalies. A depression like a bird's footprint, found behind the portal vein, meant that the demon of epidemics was about to visit the land. The condi-

tion   ained whether the patient was going
to li   ress was laid on the appearance of the
liver   made for medical students, and some
of ti   thousands of years to astonish archaeologists with their accuracy.

Apart from studying the liver, however, there were numerous
other methods by which to forecast the progress of illnesses or
drive away evil spirits. Illness was regarded as the punishment
for sin, and so, in order to obtain a cure, the patient had first to
confess his sins to a doctor-priest. The doctor-priest, who wore
a lion mask when treating 'sin diseases', would then employ a
variety of methods in order to exorcise the demons: feathers or
wool fibres could be burnt to create an unpleasant smell; the
patient could be given compresses made from plants which had
been picked by the light of a full moon; spoilt flour or decomposing matter could be applied; alternatively, the priest could make
use of snake venom, rancid fat, urine and excrement, calf's or
pig's gall, dirt which had been swept together outside the door,
and many other substances. It appears that the medicines used
were as evil-smelling and nasty to the taste as possible in order
to spoil the demon's appetite.

The temple festivals, particularly those which took place in
spring, when nature's winter rest was over, were wild affairs.
An important role at such festivals was played by the temple
girls. They were divided into different grades: the high priestess,
the brides of god or dedicated girls, and the ordinary temple
girls. The high priestess, who was also regarded as a 'courtesan
of the gods', was there for ritual intercourse with the god-king –
in the hope that this would win the favour of the 'god of fruitfulness'. The 'dedicated girls' were reserved for the priests; they
were sterilized so that pregnancy should not interfere with their
duties. The ordinary temple girls served the needs of the town's
inhabitants and those of the many strangers who were staying in
the town for the festivals.

Thus homage was rendered to the goddess of love, lust and

fruitfulness; the general promiscuity must have been indescribable. The inhabitants of Mesopotamia were, in any case, extraordinarily liberal in sexual matters. They did not believe there was any need for privacy; couples could be observed in streets and squares, gardens or fields, making love without any trace of shame. Love-boys were at the disposal of homosexuals.

These archaic sexual customs may seem surprising in a people who were, in other respects, so highly civilized. The objects found in the King of Ur's burial chamber – the golden statues of animals, head decorations and gold inlay-work, lapis lazuli and tortoiseshell, dating back four and a half thousand years – could not be made more beautifully or aesthetically today. Perhaps the sexual customs go back to the primitive forerunners of the Sumerians – those people who, in many respects still rooted in New Stone Age usages, had already settled in the land between the two rivers thousands of years before the Sumerians came.

Anyone who is interested in the history of medicine will find the emancipated way in which sexuality was worshipped interesting for another reason. If syphilis had already existed in those days, as is still assumed by one or two medical historians, then there would scarcely have been one person in the Middle East to escape catching this affliction.

The clay tablet mentioned earlier, which contains the medical text from Nippur, proves how wrong it is to assume that medical practice in Ancient Mesopotamia consisted only of magic, the black arts, devil-worship, invocations and other mumbo jumbo. Anyone living in Ancient Mesopotamia, who wanted to devote himself to medicine, had to have a precise knowledge of all the magic formulae and incantations which were used for the different illnesses, as faultless recitation of them was essential in bringing about a cure. A rudimentary knowledge of anatomy and surgery was also necessary, as well as an acquaintance with the effects of all the different known remedies. The Ancient Mesopotamians also knew how to make a kind of soap thousands of years before soap factories were thought of in the civilized countries of

Europe. Ashes of plants noted for their soda content were mixed with fats and the result was an ointment of a soapy nature. When, in about the thirteenth century BC, the Assyrian kingdom gained supremacy in the land between the two rivers, surprisingly modern ideas and a sometimes quite remarkable gift for observation turned up in Mesopotamian medicine. These were to be found side by side with the belief that diseases were brought by the gods and demons, and must be banished by means of incantations and sacrifices. Assyrian doctors knew there was a connection between some general illnesses and some dental diseases; that the appearance of plague was preceded by a mass-death of rats; they suspected the connection between mosquitoes and several different kinds of fever, and even the infrequent appearance of oriental boils, whose virus is transmitted by flies, established the belief that the flies were identified with harmful demons. The doctors also knew the clinical aspects of tuberculosis, pellagra, pneumonia, jaundice, inflammation of the gastric mucosa, intestinal obstructions, strokes, abscesses of the middle ear, lithiases and urogenital diseases.* They knew, too, that cancer of the breast was a destructive illness.

Massage, packs, bandages and compresses were commonplace and a whole range of different surgical instruments, uncovered in Nineveh, were used for the removal of a square piece of bone in skull trepanations, although the actual reason why the operation was undertaken is not known. Moreover, Mesopotamian doctors certainly carried out operations for cataract using bronze needles as long ago as 2000 BC. Catheters also have been found. Most surprising of all seems the extensive pharmacopoeia. Enemas, suppositories and advice on diets completed the medical panoply. Everything that we now know about those Ancient Mesopotamian doctors demonstrates that, in addition to a mass of demon-worship, magic and enchantment, those ancient practitioners also developed thoroughly rational methods of treating illness.

*Diseases affecting the urinary and genital tracts

During the sixth century BC, Babylon, one of the oldest, most beautiful and wealthy cities of the ancient world, was conquered by the Persians. Her civilization can be traced back thousands of years to that of the Sumerians and, at its peak, Babylon sheltered a million inhabitants within her walls. The Persians spared the city, whose hanging gardens are counted among the seven wonders of the world; and so, about a century later, when the Greek traveller, historian and geographer, Herodotus (born 490 BC in Halicarnassus, in Turkish Caria) visited Babylon, he was able to set down his impressions for posterity.

If the description of Mesopotamian healing found on the ancient clay tablets is compared with what Herodotus has to say about it, his account seems very strange. He wrote: '... having no use for physicians, they carry the sick into the marketplace; then those who have been afflicted themselves by the same ill as the sick man's, or seen others in like case, come near and advise him about his disease and comfort him, telling him by what means they have themselves recovered of it or seen others so recover. None may pass by the sick man without speaking and asking what is his sickness.'

This piece of information from the 'father of history' is hard to understand. Could everything which the people of the Tigris/Euphrates had possessed in the way of medical knowledge and equipment have been lost and forgotten during the two thousand years before Herodotus, leading him to say: 'They have no doctors'? That seems highly unlikely. It is more probable that Herodotus' report was not accurate in all points. Other descriptions by the Greek historian have also been known to depart from the truth – in some cases quite considerably. For example, Herodotus, who had a certain love of exaggeration, said that the wall surrounding the city of Babylon was about 57 miles long, 81 feet thick and 325 feet high. When, at the beginning of the twentieth century, the city of Babylon was excavated by German archaeologists, an entirely different set of measurements was revealed. The wall surrounding the city proved to have been about five-and-one-third miles long; the strongest walls were 13 feet thick and, if they had been 325 feet high, they would have had to have had much broader and stronger foundations than were found!

3

*The Egyptian, Imhotep, became the
symbolic embodiment of virtue of the
medical profession two thousand years
before Hippocrates. Numerous specialist
doctors each dealt with a separate part of
the body in Ancient Egypt. The papyri
containing medical texts.*

As darkness begins to fall over
the Nile Valley, someone taking the white sleeping-car train which
leaves Cairo for Luxor each evening will be given an unbelievably
splendid and impressive view of the kingdom of the Pharaohs.
While the golden glow of the western sky rapidly changes into
a blazing crimson, the ancient burial grounds of the Nile Valley
civilization pass like shadows in the distance. Framed by the sil-
houettes of the date palms, the gigantic phantom triangles of the
pyramids – Cheops, Chephren and Mycerinus – stand out in the
last red glow of the sun and, a little later, nearer the railway
track and visible for miles, appears the most ancient structure
of all: the two hundred-foot, six-storey high, stepped pyramid
of Saqqara.

The site on which it stands bears the traces of the most ancient
Egyptian traditions; for the history of Egypt prior to Pharaoh
Zoser, who built this first great royal pyramid – the earliest big
stone construction in the world – is lost in the obscurity of pre-
history. Neolithic flint tools and stone weapons have been found

in limestone rocks and crevices; and the bones of buffaloes, aurochs, wild asses and hippopotami have come to light in nearby caves. Doubtless the most ancient ancestors of the Egyptians were hunters; however, after the last Ice Age had retreated, when the climate became drier and the big animals disappeared, these people had to rely on agriculture to support themselves in the floodlands of the Nile. The first evidence to come down to us of the original inhabitants proves that they already possessed a hieroglyphic form of writing in the fifth millennium BC, for the Egyptian calendar is known to have been introduced on 19 July 4241 BC.

The curtain first rises on the history of Ancient Egypt in 3400 BC, when King Menes united the two kingdoms of Upper and Lower Egypt and founded the fortified town of Memphis where they met. Memphis was to become one of the most famous, distinguished and populated cities of the ancient world. Memphis reached its peak as the political centre of Egypt during the period of the Old Kingdom, which dates from about 2980 to 2475 BC. Pharaoh Zoser was born in this 'city of the white walls'; not surprisingly he ordered that his tomb, the stepped pyramid, should be erected not far from his birthplace.

The man whom he commissioned to build it in about 2800 BC must have been an all-round genius by our standards; he was an architect, a versatile scholar, poet, artist, astronomer, priest, master of ceremonies, administrator, reader to the king – and doctor. His name, Imhotep, means literally 'giver of inner peace'. Imhotep is the first doctor figure to emerge in clear outline from the shadows of history; what history tells us about him establishes him as one of the most model members of his profession. He combined wisdom and constant helpfulness with kindness of heart; the great value which the Pharaoh and his people placed on him outlasted his lifetime and caused Zoser to have his gifted vizier buried near his own tomb in the necropolis of Memphis. However, the people venerated him so much that a temple was built over his grave and, year after year, the sick came on

33

pilgrimage to be cured. As time went on, Imhotep came to be regarded as a god: this doctor, who had shown in his work such a perfect combination of wisdom and humanity, became the Ancient Egyptians' god of healing almost two thousand five hundred years before the birth of the great Hippocrates of Greece!

The Roman writer, Gaius Secundus Plinius, who compiled a thirty-seven-volume work *Historia Naturalis* (natural law) and who died during the eruption of Vesuvius in AD 79 (which destroyed Pompeii and Herculaneum) referred to Egypt as the 'mother country of diseases'. This description could also be applied to the preceding millennia, for a thorough examination of countless thousands of mummies, skulls and skeletons from the graveyards of Ancient Egypt shows that the inhabitants of the Nile Valley were, from earliest times, plagued by an excessive number of illnesses, some of which we would almost certainly designate 'ills of civilization' today.

Arthritis was an extremely common complaint; inflammation of the periosteum and osteomyelitis have also been found in countless skeletal remains. Cases of spondylarthritis or spinal deformation have been found in skeletons which are known to date from about 2700 BC. Moreover the Egyptians are known to have been afflicted with spinal tuberculosis, and also with gout and virulent osteomas. Most surprising of all, however, is probably the fact that paradentosis – tooth-root decay – which we like to blame on modern processed food, was common throughout the pyramid era, that is to say, during the first half of the third millennium BC. In addition, according to American Egyptologists who have examined thousands of skulls, caries were just as common during the early days of the Nile Valley civilization as they are today.

Even the most 'modern' of all illnesses – those concerning obstructions in the circulation of the blood – were frequently found in Ancient Egypt. Arteriosclerosis is most frequently discovered in mummies of high officials and those of the Pharaohs themselves.

Tutankhamen and Ramases V both died of a heart infection, as the English doctor, Peter Gray, was able to establish when he examined X-rays of the mummies of these two Pharaohs. This fact of medical history confirms the theory that it is not only restlessness and worry which encourage complaints of this kind but also dissipation, gluttony and lack of physical exercise. Stomach and intestinal troubles, appendicitis, gall-stones and kidney stones were not uncommon; the worst toll, however, was exacted by the infectious diseases – especially among the poorer sections of the community living in primitive conditions. The same plagues which were to afflict the inhabitants of the Nile Valley in succeeding millennia also raged in Ancient Egypt: plague and cholera, smallpox and leprosy, typhus and amoebic dysentery, malaria, tuberculosis and, not least, that 'Egyptian eye disease' caused by a virus – trachoma – which so often led to blindness.

Particularly widespread, and especially prevalent among farm workers was the parasitic disease, *schistomiasis haematobium*, which produces a tormenting type of nettle rash, pelvic pains, haematuria, stones, anaemia and general physical decline. The kidneys of some mummies have been found to contain the calcified eggs of the parasite that causes this disease. The parasite's larva are found in pools, lakes and slow-moving rivers. When it meets a human being, such as a swimmer, a labourer working in a flooded field or irrigation ditch, or a naked child at play, it bores under the skin. The cause of this multifarious disease which has attacked the inhabitants of the Nile delta for thousands of years, was only discovered in 1852 by the German doctor, Theodor Bilhartz. Since then the disease has been called Bilharziasis.

How did the Ancient Egyptian doctors combat the manifold epidemics which raged through their country? Their medicines were, like those of the Mesopotamians, the privilege of the mighty priestly orders; the doctors were priest-healers, who received their training in temple schools. As in other early civilizations, demons and spirits, magic and invocatory charms played an important part. The colossal pantheon of the Ancient Egyptian gods is explained by the fact that a different god was responsible for almost every part of the human body and also for every illness. As each healer-priest specialized in the service of a certain god, so he also had to undertake to devote himself to the illness which this god visited upon mankind.

In fact, four thousand five hundred years ago, in the days of the pyramids, there were already regular specialists. This practice was apparently maintained until the fifth century BC, when Herodotus, the Greek historian, made the following report based on personal observation of the habits and way of life of the Egyptians: 'The practice of medicine is so divided among them, that each physician is a healer of one disease and no more. All the country is full of physicians, some of the eye, some of the teeth, some of what pertains to the belly and some of the hidden diseases...'

We now know that there were specialists for all the different parts of the body more than two thousand years earlier: eye doctors, nose doctors, doctors for the upper respiratory tracts, for the 'body juices', for stomach, bladder, for baldness and premature greying. There was even a specialist on the royal anus! The Ancient Egyptians were also familiar with dentistry as is proved by those skulls in which have been found loose teeth fastened by gold wires.

The papyrus scrolls on which the Ancient Egyptians had, since their earliest days, been setting down what they knew about mathematics and surveying, the movement of the sun and stars, their stories and poems, their religious and medical texts, were less durable than the clay tablets of the Ancient Mesopotamians. But, because circumstances were favourable and the Egyptian climate helped to preserve them, many papyrus scrolls – among them quite a number on medical subjects – have come down to posterity. The deciphering of the hieroglyphics would, it is true, have taken much longer if a lucky accident had not intervened. In 1798–89 during the time of Napoleon Bonaparte's abortive

Egyptian campaign, an unknown young soldier in the pioneer corps was repairing the ruined fortifications of the redoubt Rashid near the town of Rosetta, on the western branch of the Nile estuary, when he found a slab of black basalt as big as a table-top, one side of which was polished. This stone was inscribed with three columns, each in a different form of writing. The credit for deciphering this hieroglyphic language is due to a French language expert called Jean-François Champollion – who, when only thirteen years old, was studying not just Greek and Latin, but also Syrian, Arabic, Chaldean and Coptic, the most ancient form of the Egyptian language. His appointment, at the age of nineteen, as professor of languages at the university of Grenoble provided, in the words of C. W. Ceram 'the key to all Egypt's locked doors'.

For the medical historian this meant that now the way lay clear to deciphering those papyrus scrolls which dealt with medical matters. Egyptologists from many different countries were able to continue the work so brilliantly started by Champollion and tell the waiting world what Egyptian medicine was like thousands of years ago. To the surprise of the medical specialists it was disclosed that in spite of being interspersed with details of beliefs in gods and demons, magic spells, incantations, amulets and voodoo, very serious attempts had been made to create a rationally organized doctrine of medicine. Side by side with medical papyri in which magic spells, conjuration of spirits and incantations far outnumber factual observations, there are those with pronounced empirically rational contents.

One of the most instructive papyrus scrolls of this latter kind and, at the same time, one of the oldest known handbooks of Egyptian medicine (especially with regard to what we would call accident therapy) is the Edwin Smith papyrus. This scroll, which was found in a grave near Luxor in 1862, is a copy which was probably made during the middle of the sixteenth century BC; Egyptologists assume, however, that the original dates back to the time of the pyramids, i.e. between 3000 and 2500 BC. This papyrus discusses all the measures that were taken in the care of injuries thousands of years ago: the treatment of wounds by sutures and plasters; the placing of broken bones into splints made from hollowed-out ox bones; supporting straps made of bandages soaked in quick-setting resin; the laying of flesh on wounds; cauterization and many other methods of treatment. On the other hand, the most important instrument in modern surgery – the knife – is not mentioned; therapy was conservative. Their knowledge of the skeleton was good, that of the internal organs – in spite of the prevalent practice of embalming – was deficient. The superficial structure of the brain was well known, also the fact that injury to the brain could affect parts of the body far removed from it. The brain was not, however, recognized as the seat of reason. The Ancient Egyptians rightly observed that the pulse-beat was somehow connected with the heart-beat; but the existence of the circulation of the blood – which, as we shall see, was probably suspected by the Ancient Chinese during the middle of the third millennium BC – remained hidden from the Ancient Egyptians.

A medical papyrus which has become almost better known than the Edwin Smith one is the Ebers papyrus which the German, Georg Ebers, bought in 1873 from an Arab in Luxor and which, in the opinion of Egyptologists was written, at the latest, around 1555 BC but is, once again, a copy of various older texts. Surgery, the science of the internal organs and the science of medicines, are dealt with and it is just as amazing to observe that almost nine hundred medical prescriptions existed as it is to find that many of the medical substances are still in everyday use: fennel, senna leaves, castor oil, gentian, mandragora, mandrake, henbane, hemlock, squill, thorn-apple, poppy-juice (for soothing crying children) and countless other drugs. Among animal substances still in the modern pharmacopocia, were Spanish fly (*Cantharides*), and both goat and goose fat. Several distasteful substances such as urine, excrement, fly dung and the like were also included in the Ancient Egyptian dispensary, though it is certainly too much to suppose that the users had any knowledge of the antibiotic properties of excrement and urine. It seems much more likely that they hoped to drive away the disease-producing demons by the application of these nauseating products. Among the minerals used in making up the many different pre-scriptions were magnesium, lead and copper salts, sulphur, crushed alabaster and antimony, compounds of which were considered until quite recently to be the best remedies for worms.

Of considerable medico-historical interest is a prescription which recommended that as a treatment for certain diseases, the skin be scratched with flint chips until the blood welled out. It is doubtful whether this procedure is a forerunner of the later blood-letting or whether it served a similar purpose to the Ancient Chinese practice of acupuncture of which mention will be made later.

Whereas in the Edwin Smith papyrus the magic and invocatory formulae tend to be more in evidence (apart from magical ad-vice on how to turn an old man into a young one), in the Ebers papyrus the demonic element features much more prominently.

Yet another set of papyri describes the art of healing as prac-tised by the Ancient Egyptians: the Kahum papyrus, dating from about 2150 BC and which was found in Kahum, south-west of Cairo, contains a gynaecological text; the Hearst papyrus, a collection of prescriptions from the sixteenth century BC which is presumably partly based on the older Ebers papyrus; and the Brugsch papyrus, which was written down around 1300 BC, and which is also known as the Great Berlin papyrus. It contains ad-vice on pregnancy tests which, when they were first translated and published, justifiably caused a stir. According to this, when the Ancient Egyptians wanted to find out whether a woman was pregnant, they watered wheat and barley corns with a sample of her urine and, depending on the effect, decided on the exis-tence or otherwise of a pregnancy. This procedure, which was indulgently derided as mumbo jumbo when the papyrus was first deciphered, no longer seems 'magic' to us today, for we know that considerable amounts of female sex hormone and pituitary hormone are to be found in the urine of a pregnant woman and that these active substances can very well have a lasting influence on the germination, growth and ripening of plant forms.

The Ancient Egyptians even went so far as to predict the sex of the expected child. The relevant procedure was tested some time ago by Dr J. Manger at the Pharmacological Institute of Würzburg University, who obtained surprising confirmation in many respects. It turned out, for example, that in most cases the urine of those who later gave birth to girls had produced a quicker rate of growth in the barley as opposed to the wheat, whereas a normal or even delayed rate of growth in the barley pointed to a male infant. In fact, such experiments, made under ideal conditions, resulted in up to eighty correct predictions.

In some papyri the magical elements predominated so greatly that in the Lesser Berlin papyrus, for example, which contains an account of children's ailments and their treatment, there was even a heading 'Magic Spells for Mother and Child'. Here again we have evidence of surprisingly 'advanced' and rational methods of treatment overlapping a confused mass of demonology, magic and invocations to produce a strange amalgam in Ancient Egyptian medicine. Three-and-a-half thousand years ago, the compiler of the Edwin Smith papyrus described the relationship between the two in the following surprisingly sensible words: 'Magic spells complement the effect of medicines and medicines, on the other hand, support the effect of incantations.' That is a tenet which – *mutatis mutandis* – is still completely valid in medical practice today.

4

*According to the teachings of Ancient
Chinese pathology, illness develops as a
result of alienation from the natural
order of the universe. First intimations of
the circulatory system of the blood. The
study of the pulse and glossology.
Acupuncture.*

The early history of Ancient
China is lost in the mists of antiquity. Legend tells of three
emperors, who are said to have lived during the first half of the
third millennium BC. All three, the legend relates, were not merely
rulers but also scholars, doctors, discoverers and inventors; all
three took a high measure of interest in physiological and medical affairs. The oldest of them, Fu Hsi, who is said to have lived
around 3000 BC, is supposed to have put forward the view that
every event is the result of antagonism between two opposing
moving principles. One of these, Yang, is the masculine, illuminating, creative, firm, constructive principle; the other, called
Yin, is the feminine, soft, receptive, dark and empty one. Man's
health depends upon the existence of harmony between both.

The next emperor, Shen Nung, so the legend says, was born
around the year 2820 BC and died about 2697 BC. According to
tradition, he studied the human intestines and their functions
with true passion and, in particular, the action on the body of a
variety of herbs. It is said that he had a transparent stomach and

41

abdominal wall and so could observe everything that happened inside his abdomen; so he was able to make numerous experiments with poisons and their antidotes until he was gathered to his ancestors at the age of one hundred and twenty-three.

Huang-Ti was the third legendary emperor. He only managed to live to the age of a hundred and is said to have reigned over the Middle Kingdom from 2697 to 2597 BC. Among other discoveries, he is credited with the invention of the Ancient Chinese system of pathology according to which illness is the result of alienation from the natural order of the universe. He studied the influence of the weather on the human body and is thought to have been the author of the famous book, *The Theory of the Body's Interior*, known as *Nei-ching*. This work, which was later furnished with detailed examples and commentaries, dealt with all the branches of medicine; surgery, it is true, was given pretty niggardly treatment. All discussion of Ancient Chinese pathology, however, culminates in the view that it is the doctor's chief task to restore his patient's natural balance which has been disturbed.

The *Nei-ching* is also of great medico-historical interest as it contains the very first intimations of a dawning awareness that blood circulates round the body. However, according to this book, there were thought to be two kinds of blood: one corresponding to Yang, the other to Yin. All blood was said to flow through the body in a constant stream: 'The river of blood traces a circle and never ends...' Considering the extremely limited knowledge of anatomy possessed by the Ancient Chinese, this statement seems astonishingly prophetic.

As has already been stated, the stories which have been handed down regarding these Ancient Chinese emperors are only myth or legend. Legend and folklore do not give way to history until the middle of the second millennium BC when the Shang dynasty began, that same Shang dynasty which was to remain in power for nearly five hundred years. The capital city of the Shang emperors was An-yang, which lies south-west of Tientsin near the foothills of the Tai-hang mountains on the plain of the Huang-ho.

If the ancient peoples of Mesopotamia wrote on clay tablets, and the Ancient Egyptians on papyrus scrolls, the Ancient Chinese recorded their texts on bones and sometimes even on strips of bamboo. The discovery of such bones has been informative in many ways. First, they show that, just as in all other early civilizations, religion, priestcraft, magic and a belief in demons existed in close proximity to each other, for the inscribed bones served the purpose of oracles, by means of which the priest-doctors could consult the gods about a wide variety of infirmities. Illnesses of the head, the sensory organs, the limbs, the intestines, the kidneys and bladder were described. Infectious diseases and epidemics also took up a lot of room on the oracle bones. These plagues must, therefore, as in later periods, have afflicted the inhabitants of Ancient China during the second millennium BC.

Magic and demonology also held sway over the Chou dynasty which followed the Shang dynasty from about 100 BC and continued in power for nine hundred years. Knowledge of anatomy was still extremely modest since – clearly because of ancestor-worship – the dissection of corpses was strictly forbidden. Nevertheless, a report has come down to us of one dissection of a prisoner's body during the middle of the twelfth century BC, but this must have been an isolated case for the subsequent ideas put forward by Chinese doctors about the inner organs and their functions are more or less based on speculation: five 'firm' organs, serving as collecting stations and reservoirs were thought to lie opposite five 'hollow' organs whose task was evacuation. In addition, Ancient Chinese teaching assumed the existence of so-called 'warmers', some of which were supposed to lie in the breast and some in the lower abdomen. Franz Hübotter, a doctor of medicine and an eminent expert on China, believes the term 'warmers' to refer to the lymph-ducts. The 'firm' or 'chief' organs were the lungs, liver, spleen, heart and kidneys, amongst

43

which the heart and liver were considered the most important. According to the ancient medical work *Nei-ching* (see paragraph three of this chapter) the heart was the seat of wisdom and judgement as well as of the spiritual faculties; and in view of the fact that our everyday idiom transfers a mass of psychic associations to the heart, no one should laugh at this belief. The liver and lungs were considered to be the seat of the soul and therefore, probably, the passions, just as we nowadays see a connection between the autonomic nervous system of the intestines and the emotions. Nothing was said about the spleen. Neither did the Chinese doctors know that the kidneys were necessary for the elimination of water. In fact, a man's right kidney was regarded as the storehouse of the sperm, and a woman's was supposed to have an important connection with maternity. Since the kidney's activities with regard to the secretion of urine were not known, the ureter leading from the kidneys to the bladder was completely overlooked. Water elimination was thought to take place at those places where the small intestine touches the bladder, with the water passing through the intestine wall into the bladder. The 'hollow' or 'helping' organs, in contrast to the firm ones, were the stomach, small intestine and colon, bladder and gall-bladder.

Nevertheless the practice of medicine in Ancient China advanced considerably during the Chou dynasty which lasted until 221 BC, that is to say about the time when in Ancient Greece the Macedonian victory at Sellasia ended the political significance of Sparta and when Ancient Rome was about to fight the second Punic War. What we would consider a fairly modern regulation was already in force, in that every doctor had to sit a state examination before he could practise. The most famous of all Ancient Chinese doctors, Pien Ch'io by name, also lived during the time of the Chou dynasty, that is between 500 and 600 BC. Tradition has it that he practised his art while wandering about the country. He was particularly experienced in the treatment of women's and children's diseases. Pien Ch'io is regarded as the author of the famous medical work *Nan-ching* (not to be confused with the *Nei-ching* of earlier days). It was he, too, who founded the extremely complicated old Chinese system of sphygmology, according to which a doctor was supposed to be able to diagnose an illness solely by the condition of the pulse. It was not just a question of whether the beat was strong or weak, regular or uneven, but pulses could also be distinguished as 'sounding like a sickle, first exuberant then dying away'; 'flowing along quietly like flying hair or feathers'; 'beating deep and strong like a thrown stone'; 'sounding delicate like the string of an instrument' or 'slipping along like a fish or a piece of wood on the waves'; other pulses might be 'slippery like a string of pearls gliding through fingers'; 'sunk deep like a stone thrown into water'; 'loose and slow like a willow dancing in a spring breeze' and there were those which could be said to 'swing to and fro and limp' or to 'scuttle away or stand still like a knife scraping bamboo'. From the above selection of possible pulse beats it is easy to see with what extraordinarily sharpened sensitivity the Ancient Chinese doctor examined his patient.

The classification of people who, in Pien Ch'io's view, cannot be treated, seems extremely shrewd and sensible. This includes, among others, those vainglorious and arrogant people with whom no conversation is possible; those who value their money more than they do their bodies; those who are addicted to overeating and dissipation; and, finally, those patients who believe more in magicians and enchanters than they do in doctors. Every general practitioner will instantly recognize that these classifications are still completely valid today – two-and-a-half thousand years later.

The Chou emperors helped to bring about the dangerous decentralization of China by permitting the rapid increase of feudalism. This was brought to an end by a more powerful emperor Shi Hwang Ti, the builder of the Great Wall of China which protected that mighty land from the northern tribes of barbarians. Under his successors, the Han emperors, who reigned over the Middle Kingdom for more than four hundred years, a powerful revival of Ancient Chinese medicine developed. The system of sphygmology underwent still further refinement: the patient's pulse had to be taken at eleven different parts of the body and there were no less than fifty-one different types of pulse. This over-exaggerated use of a thoroughly useful and important diagnostic device bears some resemblance to the type of 'optical diagnosis' almost entirely practised by quacks. Thirty-seven ways were known, in which the appearance of the tongue changed as a result of various illnesses. Acupuncture was also developed into the extraordinarily complicated system which is still practised by some doctors in the Western world as well today. Acupuncture is based on the theory that for every internal organ there exists a zone on the outer surface of the body where that organ's pain is felt. These areas of skin are called Head's zones after the English neurologist, Sir Henry Head, who first discovered this phenomenon. The late Dr Ferdinand Huneke of Düsseldorf was able to overcome all kinds of painful conditions by applying curative anaesthesia to Head's zones. Nowadays it is assumed that factors which are still unknown act in conjunction with the two great nerve systems Vagus and Sympathicus.

Similar reasoning and experience could also have been the basis of the ancient procedures of acupuncture so that the task it set itself – that of making good the disturbed harmony between Yin and Yang – was carried out as required by the symptoms by sticking needles into various different, exactly prescribed, places on the body. Nine different kinds of needles were used, which were said to be the invention of Hwang Ti. There were arrow-shaped needles, needles with blunt, egg-shaped or millet-seed-shaped points; three-sided needles, needles with a hair-fine tip, and many others. Those used in most ancient times were made of flint. Later, they were made of iron, gold, silver, copper and steel. It is characteristic of the scrupulous exactitude of the Chinese that there were 388 different places on the body into which needles could be set and which were left there for five minutes to a quarter of an hour or even longer.

The choice of the right time for inserting the needles also played an important role; the weather was taken into account, as also the phases of the moon and the time of day.

Another old Chinese method of treatment called Moxa, which is a kind of burning therapy, was resurrected by the well-known surgeon from Berlin, August Bier, during the first quarter of this century. In Ancient China its application involved compressing the hairs of the plant mugwort (Artemisia) into a tinderlike wad which could be wedged into little, finger-sized rolls of paper. The roll was then set alight and held against the skin for a moment until a slight burn developed. Naturally the Moxa treatment also laid down a vast number of zones on the body where this burning therapy had to be carried out. It was chiefly used as a treatment for headaches and toothaches, migraine, gout and podagra, vertigo and unconsciousness, nose-bleeding and anaemia, abdominal pains and colics, diarrhoea and loss of appetite in children, also for many other different complaints, particularly inflammatory conditions. Obviously the Moxa treatment was regarded in the light of a so-called 'irritant' therapy which relied for its effect on certain chemical decomposing agents being released during the burning process from albuminous compounds contained in the tissue, and carried along by the bloodstream to act as counter-irritants and so produce a reversal of the condition. Although August Bier was able to achieve several cures by a modernized version of this procedure, the Moxa method never caught on in the West.

Even though some of the acupuncture needles which were used to drain pus from abscesses can be regarded as early surgical instruments, surgery was still at a comparatively primitive stage. This is hardly surprising if it is remembered that, as a result of the strict prohibition against autopsy which was still in force, knowledge of anatomy was slight. Nevertheless a surgeon is mentioned who dates from the third century BC and who apparently possessed special experience in the treatment of war injuries. In those days even trepanations were undertaken, a medicine made from aconite and Indian hemp being used as a pain-killer.

At an early stage in their history, the Ancient Chinese practised a form of protective vaccination against smallpox to which they assigned the poetic name 'heavenly blossom' and of which they recognized a great many different forms. The scabs present in mild cases of smallpox were pulverized and, for preventive purposes, blown down a little tube into the nose of the person to be vaccinated. However, this procedure was not without some danger and it was not until thousands of years later, when the English doctor, Edward Jenner, introduced immunization by means of the harmless cow-pox, that vaccination became one of our most valuable means of combating epidemics.

A surprisingly extensive number of drugs was used in Ancient Chinese medicine according to a pharmacopoeia whose sources date from the second millennium BC. The sea-grape (Ephedra), whose alkaloid, Ephedrine, is still in favour today as a treatment for asthmas and allergies, was already in use during the third millennium BC against lung diseases, coughs, respiratory disorders and inflammation of the eyes. Of the numerous other vegetable remedies in the Ancient Chinese pharmacopoeia, only the most important can be mentioned: euphorbinum, aconite, calamus, chestnut, aloe, angelica, wormwood, ginsing, vetch, bamboo, senna, clematis, spurge-laurel, fennel, gentian, nutmeg, lotus, knot-grass, pomegranate, black alder, rhubarb, castor oil, sage and ginger. As in Ancient Egypt (see page 38) poppy juice was given to soothe crying children. Fresh blood and liver were re-commended in cases of anaemia – a remedy which was not redis-covered until this century; in addition, the Ancient Chinese dis-pensary also contained a great number of substances whose thera-peutic use was obviously mixed up with a belief in magic and the black arts, such as boy's urine, sweat from the skin of toads, extracts of donkey's skin, snakes' flesh, etc. The prescription of ground-up sea-horses for goitre seems thoroughly sensible, by contrast, for the iodine content of these sea animals can very well induce an enlarged thyroid to return to its normal size. Among other inorganic substances, use was made of gypsum, chalk, mercury and sulphur.

Under the Manchu or Tsing dynasty which lasted from 1644 to 1912, Chinese medicine made little progress for, as a result of the autopsy prohibition, the most mistaken ideas about the anatomy of the human body prevailed. Yet even before this, news of the great achievements in Western medicine had penetrated to China, so that interest in Euro-American medical science grew steadily keener. Furthermore, with the destruction of the monarchical/patriarchal system of government on 12 February 1912, when the 'son of heaven' abdicated his throne and the Republic of China was established under Sun Yat-Sen, the founding of Western-style medical schools began. Unlike the two types of civilization mentioned in the preceding chapters – those of Mesopotamia and Egypt – the culture of Ancient China, and with it her medical science, still flourish; therefore the Middle Kingdom now has two systems of medicine: that founded on truly Chinese origins and the Western one. The present rulers intend that both systems shall remain equally valid. In Peking there is an Institute of Ancient Chinese and Modern Medicine; whoever falls ill and is sent to hospital can himself decide, of his own free will, whether to be treated by the old Chinese folk methods or in accordance with Euro-American principles.

5

*A highly-developed sense of hygiene in
Ancient India. The Vedic and Brahmin
science of medicine. Anatomy and
surgery reached a higher level of development in Ancient India than in the other
ancient civilizations.*

Our ideas about the Indian sub-
continent's early history have undergone a radical change since
the Second World War. In descriptions as recent as the end of the
1920s, we read that no source material exists for India's earliest
history and that the only event which is to some extent certain
is the death of Buddha in about the year 480 BC. Yet it is known
that as long ago as 500 BC, tribes of foreign invaders from the
mountainous lands to the north-west, who called themselves
Aryans or 'nobles', moved into the lower-lying fertile river valleys
in a constant stream and mingled with the resident population
groups and with their civilization. Out of this union of conqueror
and subject people attached to the soil, there grew a high civilization which was most fully developed in the lands on the banks
of India's longest river, the Indus, which flows from beyond the
Himalayas in the north-west of the sub-continent down through
the Punjab into the Arabian Sea.

This Indus Valley civilization, according to most recent discoveries, reached its peak around the year 2000 BC. The cities
of that time, which were excavated after the Second World War,

bear witness to the surprisingly highly developed system of hygiene which far surpasses any similar arrangements brought to light in Egypt and Mesopotamia. Tiled drainage canals and drainpipes carried away waste water and excrement; magnificent bathing establishments, whose swimming pools survived undamaged for four thousand years, steam baths, changing and rest rooms, show the highly civilized level which had been reached in those far-off times. Certainly it would not be wrong to assume that in that era there existed, too, a well-developed system of medicine; for a high standard of hygiene, as the other early civilizations show, always goes hand in hand with a high standard of healing.

About the middle of the twentieth century BC, the Indus Valley kingdom, that thousands of years earlier had anticipated so many of the hygienic achievements of our own day, began to decline. Light-skinned Indo-Germanic invaders were responsible. They called themselves 'Hindu' (from 'Shindu', the ancient name of the Indus) and, coming from the north, penetrated into the river valleys of the Indus and Ganges. The Vedic era begins in about 1500 BC with the intermingling of dark-skinned inhabitants and light-skinned invaders, and owes its name to the Veda, the four holy Sanskrit books of the Indians, which represent the earliest record of Indian literature to come down to us. Originally created for oral transmission, they were only later written down, a task which was completed about five hundred years before our own civilization began. Their origins, however, go back two thousand years before Christ or even further, into the days before writing existed.

The Veda are of especial interest to the history of medicine because, as the oldest Indian literary monuments, they transmit the earliest information about the diseases of Ancient India and their medical treatment. Once again, a belief in magic, fear of devils and invocations are to the forefront; once again we encounter the view that disease is a punishment for sins committed and confession is a healing measure.

From time immemorial India has been the land of the great plagues, so it is not surprising that epidemic diseases such as malaria, bubonic plague, cholera, leprosy and smallpox play an important part in the ancient texts. Moreover, though they may be permeated with religion and devil-worship, the Vedic books provide evidence of the existence of a highly developed science of healing in Ancient India. The Vedic doctors knew about many healing herbs, they knew how to cauterize wounds and cases of snake-bite, they used an instrument like a catheter to treat cases of urine retention and they even constructed artificial limbs and eyes.

A further text, although similarly filled with magic and witch-craft, contains descriptions of tuberculosis, rheumatism, arthritis, epilepsy, the swellings of elephantiasis, dropsy and numerous other afflictions, as well as the plagues of tropical infections. Most of all, however, medical history shows time and time again that the doctors of Ancient India, despite a slender knowledge of anatomy, were extremely interested in surgery; and many years later their skill in this branch of healing was to perfect itself in an unexpected way. From their ancestors who had built the previously mentioned towns in the Indus Valley with such splendid sanitary arrangements, the Ancient Indians preserved their belief in the cleansing power of bathing in water,

The Vedic era of Indian medicine continued until about 800 BC. It was superseded by the Brahmin era, which was to last until the end of the first millennium AD. This era is named after the caste of wise men, or Brahmins, who determined the whole cultural trend and, with it, that of medical science. The word Brahma represented the ever-present, godlike, true and unchanging essence of all things, the world-soul; this all-one essence was, above all, inherent in the priestly man, the Brahmin. The doctors stood far below them – below even the caste of warriors – and they were awarded none of the usual honours.

Perhaps it is thanks to this in itself disagreeable circumstance that the doctors were not trained in temples and schools of

52

priesthood but had to pass through regular years of apprentice-ship. Such a training, based on practical experience, necessarily meant that the science of healing was predominantly organized on a rational basis. A student's apprenticeship lasted from his twelfth to his eighteenth year during which time he had not only to read medical texts but also to acquire practical experience in nursing, surgical treatment, visiting patients and preparing medicines.

There are many indications that, during the last centuries before Christ, the Indian and Greek systems of medicine exerted a cross-fertilizing effect. In the works of Hippocrates there is men-tion of Indian drugs; moreover, the assumption that the health of an organism depends on a balance being maintained between the three fundamental physical elements – air, mucous and bile – re-minds one of the tenets of Ancient Greek medicine. Furthermore, Alexander the Great's expedition to India, between 327 and 325 BC, created additional points of contact between India and Europe.

During the first centuries AD, medical knowledge in Ancient India attained glittering heights and the position of doctors, which had once been so low, now acquired great prestige. Three doctors stand out in particular: Charana, who lived at about the beginning of the Christian era; Susruta, who practised about five hundred years after Christ's birth, and Vaghbata, who lived dur-ing the seventh century AD. All three have left behind written works which are counted among the classics of Brahmin medi-cine; however, it is significant that the doctors themselves declare that their ideas are based on ancient Vedic traditions.

For a long time there was disagreement among antiquarians about the exact period when the Charana and Susruta works – which can be described as the oldest Indian textbooks on medicine – came into being. Then, in 1889, in the Tarim basin, east Turke-stan, local traders found an ancient Buddhist manuscript consisting of more than fifty pages of birch bark. A year later the traders sold the document to an Englishman, Colonel Bower, and, as a result of a translation made in Calcutta by the Sanskrit scholar, Dr Hoernle, it was possible to discover the dates when the ancient Indian medical texts had been written.

As in the medical sciences of other ancient civilizations, the great number of plants used for medicinal purposes is conspicuous in the Ancient Indian system, where more than seven hundred different herbs were used. In addition, there were also numerous medicines made from animal and mineral products; quite extraordinary healing powers were ascribed to mercury. Beauty preparations existed, as did remedies to stimulate virility and prolong life, and not a few of the Indian drugs found their way into the medicine chests of the Western nations. Indeed, within the last few years one of the healing plants of Ancient India – *Rauwolfia serpentina* – has acquired a high reputation in modern medicine. Its askaloid, reserpin, was rediscovered as recently as 1949, as a successful remedy for high blood pressure. The Ancient Indians also used this plant – which, because of its crescent-shaped fruit, was called 'moon plant' – as a sedative in cases of anxiety. This treatment experienced a remarkable resurrection in 1954 when it was realized that reserpin could be used to alleviate many psychotic conditions.

It has already been mentioned that of all the ancient civilizations, surgery appears to have reached its highest development in India. This implies a thorough knowledge of human anatomy and so we find that the Indian medical books of those days, in contrast to earlier times, contain regular instructions for the study of human corpses. For this purpose, corpses were steeped in water for a week to soften the tissues before the examination began. The skin was then scrubbed off with stiff brushes and the interior of the body revealed. In this way the Indians acquired a knowledge of several hundred bones, joints, muscles and blood-vessels. At that time most anatomical concepts were as confused as ideas on how the organs worked and it is therefore all the more surprising that surgery should have developed to such an exceptionally high standard. As Susruta said in his medical text-book, it demanded medical skills of the highest degree. The same medical text mentions over a hundred surgical instruments with which a great variety of sometimes quite risky operations was undertaken.

Surgical operations on the abdominal viscera were no rarity; urinary calculus was operated on by means of a lithotomy; nor were they afraid to embark on caesarean sections, being familiar with the different birth positions of a child. When the crystalline lens became dimmed, they carried out an operation for cataract, as had also been done in Ancient Mesopotamia (see page 29). Cosmetic surgery was widely practised by the Ancient Indian surgeons. Legal sentences often laid down that the wrong-doer be mutilated; for example, an unfaithful wife might have her nose cut off for adultery. The Ancient Indian surgeons would then graft a so-called 'pedunculated flap' from the skin of the cheek, forehead or upper arm to heal over the mutilated place – a procedure which has survived to this day. Straight or curved needles were used to sew up the edges of a wound. What seems to have been a most extraordinary practice was that used to close openings in the intestine resulting from operations or wounds. Large ants were placed at the edges of the wound and stimulated to bite. As soon as the wound had been clamped shut in this way, the ants' bodies were severed from their heads, leaving the teeth of the creatures behind in the organ as a fastening to the suture.

In the same way as surgery was highly developed in Ancient India, so was the knowledge of many different illnesses; the methods used for diagnosis, which included recourse to all five senses, were thorough and well conceived. No fewer than 1,120 different diseases were known to the Ancient Indian doctors. They were familiar with diabetes, which they recognized by the sweet 'honey' taste of the patient's urine; they knew that a haemorrhage from the lungs indicated consumption and that hardening of the liver was often accompanied by an accumulation of watery fluid in the stomach. But they also pondered about the causes of epidemics, which is hardly surprising when one remembers that, as mentioned earlier, India can be more or less classified as the land of epidemics. They suspected that malaria was transmitted by mosquitoes; that food contaminated by flies could bring about intestinal diseases; and they observed, quite correctly, that the appearance of bubonic plague was always preceded by a mass death of rats. As in Ancient China (see page 48), vaccinations against smallpox, with the real smallpox virus, were also undertaken quite early on in the Ancient Indian civilization.

One principle which was as highly regarded by the doctors of Ancient India, and as desirable as in our own day, was that of giving as much attention to the prevention of illness as to its cure. Accordingly, very sensible, and often positively modern, principles of health were taught, certain diets prescribed for various illnesses, breathing exercises, general cleanliness and brushing of teeth recommended. However, the rules of health did not just restrict themselves to the physical plane; there was even a regular 'psychohygiene' of rules for the health of the soul, which rested on the modern premise that without peace of mind or inner harmony there can be no true state of health.

Although it was reckoned that doctors need not bother about maimed or criminal people, nor the incurable or dying, the medical ethics of Ancient India were noticeably high. The moral code governing the practice of the doctor's profession was exemplary: 'a doctor must care for the curing of his patient with his whole heart even if his life should be in jeopardy. He may not move too near another man's wife, even in thought; he may not treat women unless their master or supervisor is present. In his clothing and general outward appearance he must be simple and modest and he must keep himself free of bad company.'

The extremely thorough and conscientious doctor's training ended with the swearing of an oath which, in several respects, resembled Hippocrates, in fact to such an extent that some people think the oath of the sage of Kios bears some kind of relationship to that sworn by Ancient Indian doctors. Especial mention was made of the doctor's obligation to preserve silence about the patient's affairs and not to tell the patient if his death was imminent; never to boast of his knowledge but to use every opportunity to extend his skills and, during examinations, to preserve all the rules of decency; always to be more solicitous for the patient's welfare than his own gain; these precepts remind one strongly of the Hippocratic oath.

Finally, during a discussion of medical ethics in Ancient India, it must not be forgotten that the establishment of hospitals took place about a thousand years earlier in India than it did in the lands of the West. When, with the prophetism of Gautama Buddha, who lived from about 560 to about 480 BC, a wave of religious fervour swept through India, hospitals were founded as a result of his teaching as they were later, during the Middle Ages, to be founded in Europe by the Christian orders. (See page 120).

As in China, a great deal of the Ancient Indian civilization has survived with the result that many of the old medical customs are still practised today, particularly those which stem from the therapeutic methods of Brahmin medicine. Because of this, modern Western-orientated medical practices are only very gradually gaining a foothold among the broader strata of people living in the Indian sub-continent.

6

The Olmek and Aztec traditions were almost totally rooted out by the conquistadores who considered them 'the work of the devil'. Extreme specialization in pre-Columbian medical science. A surprising wealth of stupefying and intoxicating drugs. The Maya in Tucatan as victims of yellow fever

The railway line, which links Vera Cruz on the Atlantic Ocean with Orizaba and Mexico City, passes a number of strange structures near San Juan Teotihuacan, about forty-five kilometres away from the capital city of the Aztecs. These structures are vividly reminiscent of the Ancient Egyptian pyramids. One of them, the Sun pyramid, is particularly conspicuous because of its huge size; and even though this edifice, with its flattened top and terraced sides on which can be seen the remains of flights of steps, may not seem as imposing as its fellows on the Nile, here, too, we must pause in amazement before the mighty work which a people accomplished with primitive tools in order to erect a worthy place of sacrifice to their gods.

Apart from this, however, they bear a remarkable similarity to the pyramids in the Nile Valley and excavations at San Juan Teotihuacan and other places have shown a striking resemblance in customs and usages, stylistic elements, pictograms and calendar composition not only to those of the Nile Valley civilizations, but also to those of Asia, for example the Ancient Mesopotamian culture. Just as there were ziggurats in Mesopotamia, so there were high temples in Central and South America before Columbus; on the other hand, several of the aspects of the Old World cultures were totally missing – for example, no trace was found of domestic animals and wheeled vehicles. Nevertheless, anyone who has seen and compared the remains of the Mesopotamian, Egyptian and Mexican civilizations, will not be able to help thinking that, thousands of years before the Spaniards arrived, some links between the Old and the New World must have existed. Indeed, the American archaeologist, Cyrus H. Gordon, has recently been able to prove that the Phoenicians reached America more than three thousand years ago.

During the first quarter of the sixteenth century, the conqueror Hernando Cortez, whose motives were reputedly not of the purest, forcibly brought the Aztec kingdom under the sway of the Spanish Crown; the terrible human sacrifices which the Aztecs offered to their gods – during which they cut the living heart from the breasts of prisoners-of-war with obsidian knives – provided a welcome excuse for the inhuman 'colonizing' activities of the foreign invaders. As the Spaniards explored the country they had conquered, they were surprised to discover the existence of a high standard of medicine in the Aztec kingdom. In a report to the king of Spain Cortez wrote that it would not be necessary to send European doctors to the New World as medical practice there was already sufficiently highly developed.

For example, the hygienic conditions in the capital of what was then Tenochtitlan, later to be known as Mexico City, were found to be far superior to those in contemporary towns of the Old World. Steam and sweating baths served for the treatment of rheumatism; a great number of medicines were stored ready for use in the pharmacies; the list of drugs used by the Aztecs was immense; they knew no less than 1,200 medical plants of which several, such as the sarsaparilla root and Chenopodium-wormseed oil, have maintained their medicinal use to this day. The Ancient Aztecs used the powdered leaves of the tobacco plant as a specific against various kinds of disease as well as for enjoyment. The conquistadores who brought back the first tobacco plants to Europe would never have suspected what a dubious gift they were presenting to the Old World.

Altogether, there is no collection of medicines in any other ancient civilization which contains quite so many narcotic and intoxicating drugs as that of the Ancient Mexicans. Of these 'magic' drugs, which were used by the ancient inhabitants of the Aztec lands to induce states of trance, three have become most widely known: the peyotl cactus, the nanakatl fungus and the seed from a species of bindweed called oluliuqui. All three pre-occupy present-day pharmacologists and doctors to a considerable degree. The secret of the peyotl cactus, in use since prehistoric times, was solved decades ago; its effective ingredient, mescalin, helped the Ancient Aztecs to reassess the whole range of their spiritual experiences. The second Aztec magic drug, the narcotic nanakatl, derived from a species of fly fungus, was used by the Ancient Aztecs because it helped them to 'hear, see and love' better. The seed of the 'magic wind' oluliuqui plant, is still used today for magic purposes by the Zapotec Indians who live in the mountainous state of Oaxaca, south Mexico, to which Christianity has scarcely penetrated.

A less dangerous endowment made by the Aztecs to the Old World was the cocoa bean. It is as hard to imagine a world without cocoa as it is to imagine a world without the chocolate which is made from it. The ancient inhabitants of Mexico, however, considered cocoa an important tonic; a strengthening drink made of cocoa, vanilla, honey and pepper was extremely popular and kept constantly available for drinking in the pharmacies. An even more useful and important gift from the ancient Mexicans was caoutchouc which, it is true, was only appreciated in Europe hundreds of years after the time of the conquistadores. The Aztec doctors, however, used enema syringes made of rubber, and prepared cantharides plasters from the juice of the rubber tree.

The specialization of doctors appears to have been as extensive as that of the Ancient Egyptians. There were specialists for eyes, dentists, specialists in phlebotomy, intestinal and bladder complaints, as well as surgeons who treated wounds by sewing them up with human hair, set broken bones, plated fractures and carried out caesarian sections. Dietary prescriptions and physical therapy were widespread and hospitals were available for clinical treatment.

From the first, it must have seemed unlikely to archaeologists that such a high standard of Aztec medicine should have been achieved by the Aztecs themselves, for they were still a comparatively young people when Cortez and his warriors invaded Mexico. The Aztecs had penetrated from the north only about four centuries before the Spanish invasion and, barbarians themselves, had taken over the civilization they found there; a civilisation which, as was learnt only fifteen years or so ago, stretched back in part to the middle of the second millennium BC, and whose origins, according to most recent assumptions, are to be found among the Olmeks on the coast of the Gulf of Mexico.

Cortez and his soldiers had no inkling of this when, after the overthrow of Mexico, they destroyed as 'magic' all evidence of a civilization which belonged to the conquered peoples and, among other things, the royal library consisting of pictograms written on scraped bark. The work of destruction wrought by the conquistadores was so thorough that only meagre relics of the medical science practised by the ancient inhabitants of Mexico in pre-Columbian times survived. Most of what we know about Aztec medicine comes from the often very extensive reports of the Spanish doctors who were sent by the king of Spain, during the sixteenth century, to Central and South America to study medical practice in the newly conquered territories.

The Maya fared no better than the Aztecs. Their kingdom was situated on the Yucatan peninsula and their chronology begins with a year which corresponds to 3113 BC by our own method of reckoning. It is true that what the conquistadores found when they reached Guatemala was only a pathetic relic of the real Maya civilization. According to the ancient pictograms, especially those of the Tizmin chronicle, which have now been completely deciphered, an epidemic of yellow fever raged among the Maya people for two centuries and it was so virulent that the greater part of the population – especially the upper stratum – died of the plague.

The fluctuating waves of yellow fever had already been weakening the ancient high civilization for almost a century; and, as they marched into the interior, the Spaniards could not but marvel at the many towns full of monumental ruins which had already been largely reclaimed by the jungle. Among them were some that had been completely abandoned and then rebuilt and re-inhabited no less than three times. Certainly, it is fairly safe to assume that it was waves of yellow fever which induced the periodic abandonment of the towns. How commonplace a calamity yellow fever in fact was, is proved by, among other things, a sign in the pre-Columbian hieroglyphic language of Central America. It represents a man with a black substance issuing from his mouth – 'vomit negro' – the black vomit, as yellow fever was called in Iberian America.

Nowadays archaeologists are again reclaiming the ancient towns from the jungle. During their excavations they have discovered that the Ancient Maya were very familiar with the art of town planning, that they knew about paper and writing, were reliably observant astronomers and made use of a calendar which far surpasses our own for accuracy. Houses have also been found which once served as steam-baths, containing hot and cold rooms; and one has every right to assume that a people who had such excellent hygienic arrangements at their disposal would also possess a high standard of medical knowledge. However, here we can only rely on guesswork for, by order of the third bishop of Yucatan, Diego de Landa, in the year 1562, all the historical books of the Maya were publicly burnt as 'works of the devil' and, as a result, the sole, irreplaceable source material about the early period of Maya civilization was destroyed for ever. Only a few scanty fragments, which can scarcely be said to deal with the Maya medical science, miraculously escaped the general conflagration and later turned up in Spain. They are now in Dresden, Paris and Madrid.

If the Aztecs are considered a comparatively young people, the same is true of the Incas who lived in Peru. They did not leave their homelands near the source of the Rio Urubamba in the Cordillere de Carabaya until the first half of the second millennium AD. They brought under their rule a widespread kingdom on the west coast of South America which, according to twentieth century archaeologists, was inhabited by a tribe which had already, two thousand years or more earlier, established its own civilization in the Mochica kingdom. The artists of this cultural era have left us a picture atlas which is probably unique: a chronicle in ceramics depicting all the events of everyday life including those relating to illness and cure. Impressive and realistic ceramics show tumours, adiposis as a result of glandular disturbances, leprosy, syphilitic symptoms, paralysis of the facial nerves, oraya fever and Peru warts (carrion's disease) and disfigurements caused by leishmaniasis of the skin and mucuous membrane, a parasitic disease transmitted by the butterfly gnat which results in an ulcerated dermal leishmaniasis similar to the oriental boil (or cutaneous leishmaniasis) but much worse.

The doctors of Ancient Peru also had a considerable knowledge of drugs. Balsam of Peru or copaiba, which is obtained from the balsam tree (myroxylon) is still in use today as is cocaine, the alkaloid derived from the leaves of the coca bush.

The medical knowledge of Ancient Peru was unquestionably superior to that of the Aztecs in the realms of surgery. Amputations were performed and artificial limbs made ending in a hollow wooden cylinder to accommodate the stump. The Incas were also active in obstetrics; they removed tumours surgically and carried out trepanations in large numbers in accordance with the most diverse, far-reaching methods – at first with knives made of obsidian and later with copper and bronze instruments. Skulls that have been found clearly show that a considerable percentage of these trepanations healed successfully.

The extent to which the Incas carried out a system of public health welfare is really astonishing and seems modern in the best sense of the word. Once a year, a big festival of health took place, in the course of which a thorough cleaning of all houses and dwellings was undertaken. Care for old people, no longer capable of work, was highly developed. Attempts were made to offer them a suitable occupation and the State was responsible for their keep. The State also looked after the lame, crippled and deformed citizens, and the fact that they were forbidden to marry seems a form of 'guided' natural selection. Their extraordinary perspicacity is borne out by the fact that they undertook forceful measures to prevent the misuse of medicines and also knew how to discourage drug addiction.

But in spite of all progress in rational healing processes and outstanding hygienic conditions, the doctors of Ancient Peru did not abandon the god and demon worship, the magic diseases and invocation of spirits which were also so much a part of their medical practice. The inhabitants of the Inca kingdom, as their predecessors had done before them, kept alive the belief that the cause of an illness could be found in the sins of the patient.

7

*Old Jewish medicine laid down excellent
rules for hygiene but the prestige of
Jewish doctors was low. In Ancient Greece
the doctors' thirst for knowledge drew
them away from an involvement in magic
and witchcraft. Rational medical science
versus 'temple medicine'.*

The most unequivocal expression of the concept that illness is a punishment from God stems from the Ancient Jewish medical science of antiquity. In the second book of Moses the Lord says to his prophet: 'If thou wilt diligently hearken to the voice of the Lord thy God, and do that which is right in his sight, and wilt give ear to his commandments, and keep all his statutes, I will put none of these diseases upon thee, which I have brought upon the Egyptians: for I am the Lord that healeth thee.' (*Exodus* 15: 26)

With such a bias towards the belief that diseases were exclusively sent by God, it is obvious that doctors could only acquire a subordinate role and that patients seeking a cure would apply to the priest in the first place. Evidence of the rather low regard in which Jewish antiquity held their doctors is given, among others, by Hiob, who says: 'You, however, are lying greasers, deceitful doctors every one of you.' So Ancient Judaea did not produce any outstanding doctors; indeed the books of Moses bear witness to the fact that it was the priests who took the rules of hygiene most seriously, as well as the battle against infectious diseases, the prevention of epidemics, disinfection and isolation and, later on, became by far the superior in these departments. Particularly in *Leviticus*, the third book of Moses, there is an abundance of regulations of which several seem thoroughly practical. First, all the 'unclean' animals are distinguished, in detail, from the 'clean' ones. 'Whatsoever parteth the hoof and is cloven-footed and cheweth the cud, among the beasts, that shall ye eat. Nevertheless these shall ye not eat of them that chew the cud, or of them that divide the hoof ... of their flesh ye shall not eat and their carcase shall ye not touch, they are unclean for you.' (*Exodus* 11: 4) These 'unclean' animals included the camel, the pig, the hare and the rabbit; also the birds of prey and a number of other birds such as ravens, ostriches and owls; finally, the animals which 'creep on the earth' such as weasels, mice, toads, hedgehogs, newts, lizards, slow-worms and moles.

While some prohibitions are hard to understand, for example the inclusion of hares and rabbits among the unclean animals (unless at the time when the commandment was formulated there happened to be an epidemic of rabbit fever among the rodents), the ban on eating pork must surely have had its origin in the danger of catching trichinosis and tapeworm. Rules for women in childbed lay down the procedure of women who have given birth. Thought was also devoted to the circumcision of boys which had to take place on the eighth day after birth; those who carried out this rule little realized, as cancer specialist Karl-Heinrich Bauer has recently observed, that the Mosaic law regarding ritual circumcision has saved millions of Jews (and Moslems) from cancer of the penis or cancer of the womb, during the past four thousand years. Bauer regards this law as almost the oldest cancer preventive in existence.

Extensive regulations governed menstrual hygiene in women and the treatment of the flow, as also sexual behaviour. Detailed instructions are further given with regard to leprosy. How it is recognized, how treated, how the clothes should be cleaned

66

whether they are made of woven material or furs; how the dwelling should be disinfected; all this is fully discussed. The inside of the house shall be 'scraped within round about and they shall pour the dust that they scraped off without the city into an unclean place'. (*Leviticus* 14: 41) If, however, this is not effective, 'he shall break down the house, the stones of it, and the timber thereof, and all the mortar of the house; and he shall carry them forth out of the city into an unclean place. (*Leviticus* 14: 45)

Further chapters deal with 'bodily uncleanliness', with suppuration, with prohibitions against blood and carrion, against eating 'what was torn with beasts', (*Leviticus* 14: 15) committing adultery, or marrying close blood-relatives or having sexual intercourse with them; prohibitions against homosexuality and sodomy are also included. Meanwhile, however wisely devised and well worked-out many of the instructions seem, all are mixed up with 'burnt offerings' or 'sin offerings', and in almost every line the reader comes across that close, inseparable connection between Ancient Jewish medicine and religion, just as was the case in all other Mediterranean civilisations.

Nevertheless, what none of the ancient civilizations had succeeded in doing, neither the Egyptian, the Mesopotamian, the Chinese, the Indian nor the pre-Columbian American – that is, the separation of medicine from god and demon-worship, invocations, sorcery, magic or expiatory sacrifice – the Greeks, a comparatively small nation in the Eastern Mediterranean, managed to achieve. This decisive break was made more than two-and-a-half thousand years ago.

The new attitude actually had its roots centuries earlier. The most ancient Greek traditions regarding medicine come from Homer and his descriptions of the Trojan War in the Iliad. Those skilled in healing who took part in this war, which ended with the destruction of Troy – the ancient Iliam – in the year 1184 BC, made no use at all of magic spells and incantations. Instead, the Homeric doctors were practical men; they were appointed as

C

military surgeons, soldiers and doctors in one. Their chief function was the care of war wounds.

During the following centuries, philosophical thought was centred among the Greeks who had settled on the coast of Asia Minor and its off-shore islands. Schools of pupils and disciples grew up round an outstanding philosopher. The founders and leaders of these intellectual communities were generally also doctors. Philosophy and medicine influenced each other more than ever before and resulted in a synthesis which has not changed to this day. These men ruled out all thought of magic in their search for truth; they sought to establish the fundamental principles of natural science such as space, matter, time, motion, life, etc., by exploring these subjects with a critical mind. A gigantic revolution in human thought divides them from the rest; a thirst for knowledge, an innate struggle for reason, were the peculiarities of this new human mentality; usefulness and function were no longer the sole criteria; knowledge was sought for its own sake. Man longed to unravel what lay hidden, to learn about himself, his nature, his physical composition, his organs and his functions.

Such an attitude was quite unprecedented – above all, this urge towards dynamic thought, the attempt to explore the true connection of one thing with another, and not to be content with the comfortable explanation that, since everything derives from gods or demons, magic and invocations are the only ways to counter them. Although the earlier chapters of this book will prevent us from making the usual mistake of thinking that Ancient Greece was the cradle of all thought or medical science, it is true to say that it was in Ancient Greece that the search for knowledge freed itself from magic or priestly ties for the first time. It was here that people first began to reflect on the harmony of the world and the purpose of existence; here that they began to observe nature and themselves, trying to understand man in all his aspects, who, after all, is himself no more than a part of nature.

Many people have tried to puzzle out why such a comparatively small group of nations like the Greeks should have been chosen to originate a revolution in thought which was to be decisive for the whole future of the world. Man's history teaches us that new concepts grow most easily at the meeting-point of different civilizations. The Greeks, themselves the product of a fusion of different tribes, were, because of their situation, exposed to the most varied influences of such foreign civilizations as the Egyptian, the Mesopotamian and later, as a result of Alexander the Great's campaigns, the civilizations of India and the Orient. From each of these the Greeks acquired elements of their wealth of knowledge and it is significant that the new way of thinking should have been born on the borders of the Greek world.

Information has come down to us about one of the oldest schools of philosophy and medicine which was situated on the periphery of the Magna Graecia of those days. It was built about 700 BC in Cnidus on the far, outjutting point of Cnidian Chersonese on the south-west coast of Asia Minor, north of Rhodes. Our knowledge of what was practised there is scanty. According to tradition, however, it seems that diagnosis played a leading part. For the rest it was – in contrast to later medical schools – active in therapy and did not simply restrict its teaching to a policy of wait and see. Treatment was concentrated more on the area where the patient's pain was felt rather than on the whole of his body.

During the sixth century BC the Greeks founded a medical school at Cos, one of the Dodecanese Islands off the south-west coast of Asia Minor. This school acquired immortal fame because of the idealized image of the doctor who taught there and who will be discussed in more detail later. His name was Hippocrates.

Another medical school grew up in Croton on the Gulf of Tarentum. The names of two of the Greek doctors who taught at this school have remained with us: they are Democedes and Alcmaeon. Democedes, who travelled all over the then known Greek world, practised his profession during his travels; from Alcmaeon, who was convinced that without a knowledge of the human body an efficient medical science would be impossible, stems the first Greek textbook on anatomy. In this, the wind-pipe and the optic nerves are described and the theory is put forward that there are two different kinds of blood-vessel. Pro-phetic, also, is his theory of the brain being the seat of the mental faculties, which Aristotle was to reverse so mistakenly about a hundred years later. Alcmaeon also expressed the thoroughly advanced view that illness is brought about as a result of an imbalance between the different components of the human body. According to the teachings of Empedocles, a native of Agrigento on the south coast of Sicily, these body components apparently consisted of the 'body liquids' – blood, mucous, yellow gall and black gall – their places of origin being, it was thought, the heart, the brain, the liver and the spleen.

The lively way in which the great thinkers of Hellas tackled all the various and different disciplines of civilized life is demonstrated most conspicuously by Democritus of Abdera in Thrace, who was born about 460 BC. From Democritus stems the theory of atoms, according to which a multitude of tiny, indivisible particles spins about in space and so brings forth matter. Democritus did not confine himself to philosophy, ethics and poetry; he was also a doctor, as is evidenced by a saying of his which is so apt today: 'Men pray to their gods for health; they do not realize that they have control over it themselves. They jeopardize it by their excesses and so their greed makes them traitors to their health.' The great humanity of Democritus' philosophy is confirmed by his conviction that the best kind of happiness was one which derived from a cheerful disposition.

While in Ancient Greece a rational way of thinking, freed from magic, was gaining ground and one brilliant mind was succeeded by another in the search for true knowledge – by critical reflection rather than by reliance on the impressions of the senses – a second medical science was still maintained, a temple medicine, closely interwoven with religion – the cult of the demi-god Aesculapius.

Aesculapius, the son of Apollo and Cornis, the prince of

Thessaly's daughter, is usually represented holding a clublike staff and holy snake. He plays an important role in Greek mythology as a healer and worker of miracles. He was even able to raise the dead. His cult gained more and more ground during the fifth century BC when shrines were built in his honour at numerous places. Moreover those sites were preferred which were set in natural surroundings most beneficial to healing, whether because they were in attractively wooded mountain-country, or because of their favourable climates or healing wells.

What the city of Rome is to the Catholic Church, so Epida irus – a town opposite Athens in the Eastern Peloponnese – was to the cult of Aesculapius. As a combination of shrine, health resort and place of pilgrimage, Epidaurus had achieved a status similar to the shrine at Lourdes; despite the fact that the most ancient shrine to Aesculapius stood at Thessalonian Trikkala, it and others at Athens, Pergamon and Smyrna were regarded by the Ancient Greeks as of subordinate status to the shrine at Epidaurus.

Two thousand five hundred years later, what is left of the healing resort in Epidaurus is still able to arouse the amazement of visitors. The foundations of one sanatorium still stand; it had 180 rooms and two dormitories each about 230 feet long, at the disposal of people seeking a cure. A bathing establishment and the fifty-foot deep well of Aesculapius are reminders of all that was done for the comfort of visitors to the healing-shrine, but their cure was certainly also helped by the attractive scenery and, above all, by the healthy climate. Just as every modern spa has its theatre, so a theatre with fifty-five rows of seats and exemplary acoustics was provided for the entertainment of visitors. It is so well preserved that the tragedies of Euripides, Sophocles and Aeschylus are still performed there today.

Sleeping in the temple played an important role in temple medicine. The priests would instruct the patient to sleep near the statue of Aesculapius and it is very probable that a drugged drink was also given to him. The long journey which most of the patients had made and the patient's own feeling of credulous expectancy would tend to heighten his readiness to believe in miracles – a phenomenon that can also be observed at Lourdes.

Educated Greeks disliked the whole flavour of temple magic with its mystic-oriental impact. As the rational scientific type of medical science prospered, temple magic became more and more a matter for the lower classes. The most witty of all Greek dramatists, Aristophanes, who depicted the public life, customs and establishments of Ancient Greece with an equal measure of truthfulness and unmerciful mockery, was able to ridicule the temple superstitions and denounce the priests of Aesculapius as grasping charlatans.

When Aristophanes was born, Hippocrates was just ten years old. He was destined to become the idealized image of a doctor of all time; and the sobriquet 'the great' was not added to his name at some later date; Aristotle had already called him this. Galen describes him as 'the godly'. The Middle Ages turned him into 'the Father of Medicine', for what has been discovered today about the medical sciences of the older civilizations was totally unknown at that time. Even though we ourselves no longer believe that medical science began with Hippocrates, we cannot help but commend his outstanding new conception of the true ethics of medicine which has remained valid to this day.

8

*The 'father of medicine', Hippocrates,
creates a new style of doctor with a
standard of professional ethics that is valid
to this day. A theory of body liquids; the
concept of holism and the constitution;
one man reacts in a different way from
another. The further separation of
medicine from a religio-priestly amalgam.*

Anyone who has once seen the
island of Cos in the Dodecanese, as it nestles in a lapis-lazuli
coloured, foam-capped sea, with its ochre-coloured beaches and
towering mountain peaks, its rippling pinewoods and the dusky
cypress groves, bright plane-trees, elms, orange and lemon trees,
will never forget the sight. It was the home of the greatest doctor
ever known, the most ancient, and at the same time the most
modern of doctors, Hippocrates.

What is known about his life is fragmentary and dubious. He
was born about 460 BC, the son of the doctor Heraclides. His
mother, Phainarete, was a descendant of the family of Aesculapius,
one of the noble families of Cos, whose ancestral line, which went
back to the sixth century BC, was said to descend from the god of
healing himself.

In ancient times, Hippocrates was already thought the greatest
doctor of all times, the father of doctors, in fact the classical
originator of medical science. He received his initial training

from his father, and counted Herodicos, the Sophist Gorgias, and the philosopher Democritus of Abdera, mentioned in the previous chapter, among his later teachers. He was born in a brilliant era. Socrates was pronouncing his philosophy, Thucydides was at work on his histories, Sophocles was thrilling audiences with his tragedies, Praxiteles was creating his unique masterpieces of sculpture and Pericles was practising his brilliant statesmanship.

Hippocrates practised his profession on countless journeys through Hellas and the cures which he achieved soon caused him to become the most famous doctor in his own country, and one who was constantly called in when all other help had failed. He spent some time in Chizikos on the Propontis, also in Meliboia and Abdera in Thrace. He visited the island of Thasos and – according to tradition – perhaps even travelled to southern Russia, Egypt and Kyrenia. In 429 BC he was in Athens fighting the plague which claimed Pericles among its victims and he spent the last days of a life rich in fulfilment and blessings in Thessalian Larissa, where he died in 377 BC.

The place where he was buried has disappeared long ago, as have the details of his life story. One thing, however, remains and will live on as long as there are civilized people in the world, that is the memory of his great humanity and professional skill, his exemplary conduct, the nobility of his views and his high standard of professional ethics.

These qualities, all of which were part of his intellectual make-up, together comprised what is known as Hippocratism – the 'queen of Hellenic intellectual achievement' – and were already valued by the ancients to the fullest degree. Plato regarded him as the intellectual equal of Pheidias and Polycletus; Aristides compared his high artistry with that of Pheidias and also with the painter Xeuxis and the orator Demosthenes. Moreover, what was most admired and respected was not the medical skill itself, with its techniques and dogmas, but the whole high ethical concept of medical science together with the rational nature of its theory and practice, which have made him a prototype for doctors of all time.

He was concerned not just to treat a sick organ, but with the whole patient; his attention was always fixed on the general condition, the totality, of the sick man. For – 'The human body is a circle, of which each part may be esteemed as both the beginning and the end ... of the knowledge of their parts, their sympathy and communication. By the affection of one part, the whole body may become affected ...' (*De Locis Homine* I: i The writings of Hippocrates and Galen, abridged from the original Latin by John Redman Cox MD, 1846.) A genuinely warm humanitarian attitude is the fundamental basis on which his healing activities were built. He maintained that the chief aim of treatment was to draw observation of nature, the constitution and circumstances of life into the field of examination in support of the natural healing processes. The theory of 'body liquids' or 'humoral pathology' which, as mentioned previously, he inherited from Alcmaeon of Croton, has, as a result of the findings of modern physio-chemical research, experienced a remarkable resurrection. Similarly, the then new directions into which he channelled medical thought are those now followed in the comprehensive medical attitudes today.

Hippocrates' greatest contribution, however, was his belief in the ethics governing the practice of medicine, as expressed in the oath which the young Asclepiades of Cos had to swear before being admitted to the medical profession and in the idealistic and model way in which the doctor's code of ethics is summarized. This code has not lost its validity to this day and it is of no great importance whether every word of it derives from Hippocrates himself or whether, perhaps, as was suggested in Chapter 5, parts of it may derive from Ancient Indian influences. Integral parts of the oath were the vow to bring into play, for the good of the patient, those principles governing a way of life which were recognized as right, to the best of the doctor's knowledge and belief; to give no one a lethal medicine even if the doctor should be asked for one, nor to tell a patient how to obtain such a medicine; never to give a woman an abortifacient; always to keep his personal life and his work as a doctor pure and untarnished; to enter a house only in order to heal the sick and to avoid every conscious wrong, especially that of making advances to female persons; whatever he sees or hears during his work or learns as a result of it from other people may never be communicated but must be kept absolutely to himself in the conviction that such things are strictly secret.

Best and most lucid is the list of virtues which the philosopher of Cos – who created an entirely new type of doctor as much by the conduct of his exemplary life as he did through the quality of his work – demanded of all members of the medical profession, and which were summarized by him as: objectivity, consideration, modesty, dignity, respect, judgement, decision, cleanliness, wisdom, knowledge of all things useful and necessary to life, aversion towards evil deeds, and freedom from superstition and conceit.

It is not certain whether Hippocrates himself left any written work to posterity; of the seventy-two books which were written between 480 and 380 BC, and assembled in Alexandria under the title, *Corpus Hippocraticus* during the third century BC, it is only possible to say that they spring from the Hippocratic school and exude a Hippocratic flavour. Other doctors must surely have helped to write them down, but by connecting the work with Hippocrates' name, they assured it a universal interest.

The book *The Sacred Disease* (*De Morbum Sacrum*) confirms most unequivocally the total separation of Hippocratic medicine from any involvement with magic. It begins by saying in a downright, authoritative way:

I am about to discuss the disease called 'sacred'. It is not, in my opinion, any more divine or more sacred than other diseases, but has a natural cause, and its supposed divine origin is due to men's inexperience, and to their wonder

at its peculiar character. Now while men continue to believe
in its divine origin because they are at a loss to
understand it, they really disprove its divinity by
the facile method of healing which they adopt, consisting,
as it does, of purifications and incantations. (*The Sacred
Disease* (*De Morbum Sacrum*) Hippocrates II, transl.
W. H. S. Jones, Wm. Heinemann New York; G. P. Putnams
Sons MCMXXIII.)

The dividing line between priestly and rational healing could
hardly have been drawn more sharply. Yet in spite of all this,
the Hippocratic doctor was nothing if not god-fearing, for Hippocrates believed that 'the art of healing led to a devoutness
towards God, and love towards mankind' and 'where there was
a love of art, there was also a love of humanity.'

The *Corpus Hippocraticus* deals with different branches of
medicine. One book, entitled *About Air, Water and Places* could
be regarded as the first medical climatology, Others are devoted
to surgery. The book *About the Nature of Man* describes the
theory of body liquids in utmost detail. As mentioned earlier
this theory was based on the existence of four cardinal fluids:
blood, mucous, yellow gall and black gall. Moreover blood represented the warm-damp principle, mucous the cold-damp, yellow
gall the warm-dry and black gall the cold-dry principle. Other
fluids were the intestinal juices, lymph and semen – as had already
been taught in Ancient India. Illness was the result of a wrong
mixture of the liquids or *dykrasy*; health, on the other hand,
depended on the correct blending of the liquids, or *eukrasy*, as
a result of which the harmony of an organism was guaranteed.

The book *Prognosticon* evidently comes from Hippocrates
himself. It demonstrates a very sharp talent for observation and,
by means of accurately described symptoms, explains the prog-
noses which played an important role in Hippocratic medicine.
A feature common to all books, in spite of some contradictions,
is that they are all imbued with the Hippocratic spirit and put

professional ethics before all other medical virtues. This attitude is expressed most forcibly in *The Law* and *The Doctor.*

The strong influence which the ancient oriental civilizations had on Hippocratic medicine can be seen from *The Book on the Number Seven* (see also page 25), which is of considerable significance when considering the 'critical days' mentioned in the Hippocratic theory of medicine.

The work *About Ancient Medicine* refers in the utmost detail to the subject of diet, one of the most important Hippocratic therapeutic factors. This taught that during the summer a different diet was required from that which was wholesome during the winter; that children must be given different food from adults, and thin people a different diet from fat ones.

A sphere of knowledge which goes back to Hippocrates and on which great value is laid today is the way in which food is prepared. Moreover, dietetics were by no means only concerned with the way of eating: It was thought that food alone would not achieve health; many other things had to be added: gymnastics, strengthening exercises, baths, massage, the use of light, air and water, breathing exercises, voice exercises and many more things besides. Finally, it was believed that every case demanded its own special diet.

This dictum underlines one of the fundamental problems of Hippocratism: the attention given to the constitution which is generally described by Hippocrates as *pthisis* (nature). First the natural condition of the whole person had to be known. After that, knowledge of the effect of every different food and every different drink. Moreover, it was necessary to know their natural effect just as much as the one which they would have after the intervention of the human mind and skill. It was also thought better to try to follow nature; and watch the human constitution and human forces.

Possibly, apart from the unique code of professional ethics and the conscious detachment from religio-priestly amalgamations, the introduction of the concept of man's constitution represents the

most creative aspect of Hippocratism. High standards of professional ethics can also be found in the medical sciences of much
older civilizations (see page 56) and much higher levels of treatment by medicines, of surgery and hygiene can sometimes be
found thousands of years before Hippocrates. But the knowledge
that each man reacts differently from the next, and the intellectual
penetration of this idea, is the achievement which can be solely
attributed to the school of Cos.

This was accomplished because Hippocrates was, above all else,
an empiricist, that is, he based his method of healing on the
knowledge he had gained by his own experience. This, however,
constantly reminded him that different people's reactions to the
methods he employed varied greatly; that every man has a special
inborn force with which to combat disease in one way or another.
Hence the Hippocratic maxim: that it was not the doctor who
cured the disease, but the man's body which cured it; hence, also,
a conservative element in the treatments employed, and the humble
acceptance that it would never be possible completely to fathom
the processes governing sickness and health.

The Hippocratic doctors, being empiricists, were keenly observant; they knew just what signs indicated a dangerous turn
in the course of an illness – such as the changed colour of the
face, hollow-eyed aspect, sunken temples, pointed nose, cold ears,
etc. They used all their senses in observing a patient yet it seemed
to them that the science of healing was even more important
than the knowledge that experience had given them, or the facts
which their senses had grasped. They believed, moreover, that
the real science of healing, which seemed to them the most distinguished of all arts, could not be learnt but was inborn; it was
a natural gift, inherent in a doctor.

Even though cranial foramens were undertaken, limbs amputated,
a suppurating kidney removed, stomach operations and lithotomies
carried out, abscesses opened, cupping applied, scratches made
in the skin and even the use of red-hot irons not scorned, treat-

ments were thoroughly conservative and carefully applied. The extremely modest anatomical knowledge alone – to which, it is true, no great importance was attached – discouraged a higher development of surgery. In the same way, only a few medicines were used, and Hippocrates' saying that to prescribe nothing is sometimes an excellent medicine seems especially relevant today. Such medical substances as were used came from India or Egypt, and included henbane for anaesthetics, turpentine, juniper, cypress and laurel oil, valerian, cinnamon, wormwood and mint.

The fact that medical substances were used only sparingly is explained by the regulation of Hippocratic medicine under which it was the duty of a true doctor to support nature in her healing activities and not to undertake anything which could infringe upon or disturb this process. According to this Hippocratic concept, the doctor is the servant, the 'helper' of *pthisis*. 'It is important to help, or at least not to harm; to undertake nothing useless, but also not to overlook anything.' With these words, Hippocratists did not commit themselves either to an allopathic or a homeopathic point of view: 'It has been well established that some diseases can be brought to a fortunate conclusion by use of the opposite principle, others, on the other hand, by use of a similar one.'

In order to understand the point of Hippocratic medicine, which seems strange, and even backward to us in so many respects when compared with that of the much older oriental civilizations, it must be remembered that the Hippocratic doctor's chief concern was not diagnosis. Prognosis and therapy were disproportionately more important to him. 'His chief interest', says the medical historian, Erwin H. Ackerknecht, 'was not for the illness as such, but for the patient, or carrier of the illness. He concerned himself more with the body as a whole, than with changes in any individual part.'

This limited interest in the 'individual parts', this almost exclusive focus on the general and the whole, naturally had its drawbacks. The exploration of anatomical findings and individual organs did not stand high in the Hippocratic doctor's interest; and in Hippocratic medicine, which was certainly no specialist science but available to anyone, anatomical considerations certainly played a subordinate role.

As a result, the *Corpus Hippocraticus*, in spite of its imposing dimensions, contains only modest anatomical observations which sometimes seem rather muddled. The brain, according to Hippocratic conceptions, is a 'big gland'; true, the optic nerves connecting the eyes with the brain were known, but they were thought to contain 'sight fluid'. The Hippocratic doctors knew quite a lot about the bones of the skull, but were less familiar with the vertebrae. They made no distinction between sinews and nerves; the windpipe was a vessel which transmitted air to the lungs and heart for cooling purposes. The liver and spleen were thought to be the chief sources of blood, from where it was sent to the heart to be warmed. What is surprising is that the whitish liquid, chyle, in the intestinal lymphatic vessels, was mistaken for mother's milk. According to Hippocratic ideas, the growing uterus squeezed this 'milk' up from the stomach regions into the mammary glands.

It may seem surprising that a man of the intellectual stature of Hippocrates should lay such little stress on the actual foundations of medical science, without which we of today can barely imagine any medical treatment. However, his attitude towards his patient was fundamentally different from that of doctors today. The Hippocratist's first consideration was to be certain he was exercising his healing skill at the sick-bed and, while so doing, to take in the totality of the sick person. For 'every illness, even though it may reveal itself by means of local symptoms, is nevertheless first and always a general disease and the individual part can never be recognized without seeing the whole'.

9

*Aristotle, one of the most widely
respected of all learned men; doctor,
scientist and philosopher. With Hellenism
a new era in the history of medicine begins.
Medicine now becomes a specialist profession. Herophilus and Erasistratus
'discover' the nervous system. The focal
point of medicine moves from Alexandria,
the citadel of Hellenism, to Rome.*

It is not hard to realize that as
scientific medicine developed further, knowledge of anatomy
could not continue to remain as low in the scale of interest as it
had been with the Hippocratic doctors. So, only a short time
after Hippocrates' death, during the fourth century BC, a doctor
became famous who, by his research and knowledge, demonstrates that interest in anatomy was beginning to become more
and more active. His name was Diocles and he came from Carystus on the island of Euboea. The sphere of his activities was
not on the periphery of the Greek world as had been the case
with earlier philosophical and medical schools; instead, Diocles
practised his profession as doctor in Athens, the metropolis itself.
Valued for his amiable disposition and esteemed because of his
oratorical gifts – so important in ancient Hellas – he became
known in Athens as a second Hippocrates.

Diocles was also a much-travelled man. He wrote sixteen books but, though all the titles are known, of the texts only fragments remain. One of them deals with anatomy; Diocles, like so many anatomists of the past, apparently obtained his knowledge by dismembering various animals, and based on this his conclusions on the human organs and their functions. Nobody yet dared to venture near human corpses. In spite of his zealous studies of anatomy, Diocles arrived at the mistaken idea that the heart was the central controlling organ of the body and must, therefore, also be the seat of all mental disease. With extraordinary obstinacy this same mistaken opinion was to be maintained by his great contemporary, Aristotle.

Diocles of Carystus also wrote books about medical plants and poisons. Most modern, however, were his comments about hygiene. What he wrote about a healthy way of life has come down to us intact and deserves full attention even today, two thousand three hundred years later:

Rise before sun-up. Wash the face and head. Tooth-care
– whereby gums and teeth should be carefully rubbed with
peppermint powder. Rub oil into the whole body. Then
take a little walk before starting work. At midday visit the
gymnasium and perform physical exercises. Then have a
bath and massage. Breakfast is understandably plain: bread,
a light porridge with vegetables, cucumbers or similar
vegetable, depending on the season, everything being prepared
simply. Quench the thirst with water before eating. After
the meal, drink white wine mixed with water and a little
honey. After breakfast, during the midday heat, comes the
siesta, in a cool shady spot free from draught, as in all
southern countries. Then, back to work and later another
visit to the gymnasium. In summer, the main meal takes place
during the evening shortly before sunset. It consists of fruit,
vegetables, bread and fish or meat. The day ends with a short
walk and bed sought early.

During the lifetime of Diocles of Carystus a new star rose in the firmament of Greek science. Aristotle was born in 384 BC in Macedonia Stageira on the Chalcidice in north-east Hellas. The son of the king's personal physician, Nicomachus, he was seven years old when Hippocrates died. Like his father, Aristotle became a doctor; in addition, however, he was destined to become one of the most widely respected of all learned men, at once both scientist and philosopher. After the age of eighteen, Aristotle spent twenty years in Athens as Plato's pupil; he founded a university there and taught his puplils that – contrary to Plato's idealistic arguments – experience derived from observation is the foundation of all knowledge. Since he liked delivering his lectures while strolling through the shaded arcades (*peripatoi*) of the Lyceum, his was known as the peripatetic school. Aristotle left the then capital city of science and the arts when the Athenians declared war on King Philip of Macedon, the father of Alexander the Great.

He was forty-one years old when King Philip called upon him to become the private tutor of the thirteen-year-old Alexander. The many extremely accurate descriptions of strange animals not found in Greece would seem to show that Aristotle accompanied his royal pupil on at least some of his campaigns. At the age of fifty-three, Aristotle returned to Athens where, with remarkable productivity and diversity he produced those basic works which, on the one hand, led him to become known as the father of logic and, on the other hand, as the founder of science – the first biologist in the comprehensive meaning of the word.

Aristotle, whose teachings remained valid for hundreds and even thousands of years, believed firmly that nature never creates anything without a purpose. For him the principle held good that true knowledge, true judgement, can only be obtained by observation, experience and perception; knowledge and information were to him an end in themselves regardless of practical use or religious considerations. His *History of Living Creatures* (*Historia Animalorum*) breaks as much new ground as his book on the breeding and evolution of animals; his zoology also established the science of morphology. Aristotle taught that there is a form-giving force and passive matter; in lifeless nature, matter is higher than form; in organic nature, form dominates matter. The modern idea that certain organs, regardless of their present function, have common basic origins was already foreshadowed by Aristotle. When he compares fishes' scales with the feathers of a bird, the fins of fishes and seals with the limbs of four-footed animals, he is anticipating trains of thought which were not to be clearly stated until more than two thousand years later.

Aristotle's exploration of the human organism was hampered because religious, ethical and aesthetic inhibitions still prevented a more intensive preoccupation with human anatomy. Nevertheless, one is tempted to assume that Aristotle had not merely acquired his knowledge of the construction and organs of the human body in the same way as his predecessors, namely by applying directly to the human organism what he discovered in carefully dissected animals. From where else could he have learnt that there are quite specific peculiarities in the structure of the human heart – even though he does make the mistake of thinking that it has only three chambers.

Moreover, he demonstrates that he knows the connection between the heart and the blood-vessels and the way in which the arteries stem from the great aorta. His works repeatedly categorize together certain parts of the body which would nowadays generally be termed 'tissue', such as cartilage, bones, flesh, fibre, fat, etc. These 'similar' components he sets opposite the dissimilar or different ones. Although such a dictum as: 'Though flesh can be divided into more flesh, a hand cannot be divided into hands,' now seems obvious, in the context of those times it represented an epoch-making discovery.

In addition to so much positive enrichment of knowledge, it must be admitted that the sage of Stageira also produced some confusion in the realms of anatomy; and the worst of it was that his mistakes survived with exceptional persistency. According to Aristotle, people sleep because food causes a warming perspiration.

In general, the concepts 'warming' and 'cooling' play an important role in Aristotle's *Physiology* – for example, old age is also said to derive from a 'cooling' process. The 'hard-fleshed' people are ill-endowed, those of 'soft-flesh', on the other hand, being talented. Infants are fair-haired at first because they have eaten so little. When food reaches the heart it 'cooks' and turns into blood. The oriental-Mesopotamian influence is again demonstrated by the theory that after two times seven years the human being ripens.

One of the most fatal sources of error in Aristotle was, as mentioned before, his unswerving conviction that the heart was the 'source of life', the 'acropolis of the body' and the 'beginning of the organism'. He believed it to be the first organ to be formed as the body developed. Accordingly, Aristotle taught that the heart was the 'source of life and the seat of human intelligence'; also that the nerves emanating from the sensory organs and from the periphery of the body lead to the heart, the 'seat of the soul'.

The growing awareness of many doctors (see page 70) that the brain was the central organ which controlled the functions of all the others and was also the seat of the mental faculties was once more shaken. The brain, which Aristotle saw as 'bloodless, cold and without sensation' was demoted to a position of inferiority, namely a 'steaming gland there to cool the heart.' The idea of the heart being the source of the mind has lasted in the most persistent way for thousands of years; we still use the word 'heart' a great many times a day in connections which have nothing at all to do with the circulation of the blood.

Aristotle died in 323 BC only a year after his great pupil, Alexander of Macedon, had succumbed to a high fever, probably malaria. However, ten years before his death, Alexander the Great had founded the town of Alexandria on the Mediterranean coast of Egypt at the north-west corner of the Nile delta. This town was to enjoy an unexpectedly brilliant revival when the great military genius, empire-builder, civilizer and merger of cultures was succeeded there by the Ptolemies. Athens lost its position as metropolis, the Greek State became Hellenism which, for three centuries, was to maintain its supremacy in art and science, not least in the natural sciences and medicine. Quickly the splendid town of Alexandria became the citadel of a new science which was still based on Aristotle's teaching but in which the Greek and oriental character and knowledge merged and fertilized each other.

With Hellenism a new era in the history of medicine began. The individual disciplines started to separate one from another and medicine increasingly became a science. Homeric doctors were still methodical craftsmen; Hippocratic medicine itself had a craftsmanlike character and the Hippocratic books could be understood by any reasonably educated person. Now, however, the art of healing became a specialist science, which required specialist knowledge and found literary expression in a growing body of specialist literature.

Alexandria, with its library of a hundred thousand books, was the ideal place for the ever-growing number of medical books to collect. A new phase in medicine began, for now the Hellenistic scientists clearly recognized that only those who were familiar with the internal construction and laws governing the life of the human body could practise the art of healing. So a systematic study of anatomy was immediately introduced, and was encouraged by the science-loving Ptolemies. For the first time people did not shrink from a study of the human corpse and so at last achieved the basic prerequisite for true anatomical knowledge, the dissection of human bodies.

The highly developed Egyptian art of embalming had already provided many opportunities for getting to know the internal organs; now a systematic exploration of the human body was supported by the highest authority which made available to scientists the bodies of recently executed criminals. In his book *About Medicine*, the Roman writer, Aulus Cornelius Celsus – it is true he lived three hundred years later – mentions that the

Egyptian kings even placed living criminals at the disposal of scientists for anatomical and physiological study.

Among the scientists who were called to the Ptolomeic court in Alexandria were two doctor-anatomists, whose names are indelibly engraved on the history of medicine: Herophilus of Chalcedon on the Bosphorus, and Erasistratus who was born in Julis on the Cycladic island of Chios in the Aegean. Both were true pioneers of medicine and anthropology, and it can be said that they were the true discoverers of one of the most important systems in the body, the nervous system. Aristotle had not recognized any sharp division between nerves and sinews; Herophilus was the first to make this distinction and to discover the true characteristic of nerves as instruments of sensation. Even more remarkable, he recognized that the brain was the most important part of the nervous system and was its controlling organ. When one remembers that Aristotle's authority was regarded as irrefutable, this was no mean achievement.

Herophilus had a surprising knowledge of numerous anatomical details connected with the brain. He knew about the meninges, the cerebellum and many other parts; indeed certain areas of the brain still preserve his name in their scientific designation, He also gave an accurate description of the blood supply to certain sections of the brain, understandably so as he was a pupil of Choean Praxagoras who was probably the first person to distinguish the difference between arteries and veins. The duodenum was given its name by Herophilus and the liver and reproductive organs were accurately described in his work *Anatomics*.

Inventive though Herophilus may have been in his anatomical research, when it came to medicine, however, he continued to follow the course mapped out by Hippocrates. He, too, based his knowledge on the theory of body fluids and he further believed in the existence of four life-guiding elements: a nourishing force located in the liver; a warming one in the heart; a sensitive one in the nerves and a thinking force located in the brain. In the field of diagnostics, he developed a carefully worked-out

88

sphygmology which was almost as complicated as that employed in Ancient Chinese medicine (see page 45).

Dietetics occupied as important a place in his medical treatments as it had in those of Hippocrates; in addition, he also made copious use of medicines which he described as 'divine hands'. He was familiar with surgery and obstetrics, and even wrote a book on midwifery.

His view that the prevention of an illness is better than its cure seems highly congenial. He coined the phrase: 'Wisdom and art, strength and wealth, all are useless without health.' Perhaps Goethe knew of this dictum when he wrote: 'What use to me is gold and wealth, if I do not enjoy good health?'

A further step forward in the investigation of the human body was achieved by Erasistratus, who was only a little younger than Herophilus. He, too, added many discoveries of details valuable to the anatomical and physiological knowledge of his day. While stressing the anatomical unity of the brain, the spinal cord and the nervous system, he noticed that the cerebrum of a human brain had many more convolutions than those of the animals which he had examined; from this he drew the conclusion, which seems obvious today, that this difference is connected with man's superior intelligence and that, as a result – contrary to Aristotle's assumption – the brain must be the centre of the thought processes.

Erasistratus also gave thought to the way in which impulses registered in the brain are transmitted to the organs of the body. He imagined that the hollow spaces in the skull were filled with a 'mental air' which was passed on to the muscles by the nerves (which consequently must contain narrow channels) and gave them the impulse to contract. In all honesty it must be admitted that even today, in spite of immense advances in research, millions of experiments on animals and the use of the electron microscope, scientists still do not know a great deal more about the way in which impulses are transmitted by the nerves.

The most important discovery made by Erasistratus is un-questionably his realization that there are two different kinds of nerves: one kind which transmits sensations from the periphery of the body to the brain, which he had recognized was the centre of the nervous system; and a second which transmits the impulses from the brain to the muscular system. Erasistratus set down his discoveries in two books of anatomy; what survives of these contains – apart from the account of the brain and nervous system already mentioned – outstanding descriptions of the wind-pipe, and the epiglottis, the liver and the bile-duct, the heart and the cardiac valves.

As a doctor, Erasistratus was not so conservative as his older colleague, Herophilus. He abandoned the traditional theory of body fluids and tried, by means of anatomical study, to compre-hend localized illness; he was therefore one of the first doctors in ancient times to think along similar lines to modern physio-logists and pathologists. When he grew old Erasistratus retired to the island of Samos. However an incurable disease deprived him of his well-earned *otium cum dignitate* (leisure with dignity) and led him to bring his own life to an end. The school of Erasi-stratus was to remain active for nearly five hundred years.

As one idea gives way to another in the eternal development of thought and one extreme calls forth an opposite, so it was with Greek medicine. The more the art of healing developed into a pure science, the louder came the cry that the actual practice of healing should not be forgotten among all this research into anatomy and the nature of disease. It was rather like a contem-porary feeling of conflict between physician and medical research scientist.

Heraclides of Tarent, who lived and worked about 75 BC, seriously doubted whether for practical healing purposes, it was even necessary to know about anatomy and the construction of the human body. This philosophical scepticism, which questioned the possibility of attaining a sure and objective knowledge of reality threw its shadow over the new medical science which had calmly and sensibly based its knowledge on personal experience and was essentially organized on practical lines. Heraclides was the author of detailed books on pharmacology, a book about the treatment of internal illnesses, another about the treatment of external ones, as well as a dialogue entitled *Symposium* on dietetics. It was characteristic of the sceptics that they were not afraid to affirm a truth which has always existed, but which almost every doctor has avoided admitting, namely that making money is the purpose of medical practice.

About two centuries after Herophilus and Erasistratus had established the fame of the Alexandrian medical school, another change took place on the stage of world history. True, Alexandria continued to flourish as the nursery of the sciences, but its importance in world politics was over once Caesar had conquered Egypt; now a new star began to shine ever more brightly in the sky of antiquity. This scene changed and the centre of medicine moved, from Alexandria on the periphery of the Greek world, to the capital of the Roman Empire.

What the new sovereign of the *orbis terrarum* had to contribute to the development of medicine was modest enough, so permission was given, though occasionally somewhat reluctantly, for Greek doctors to settle in Rome. Caesar was even to grant them Roman citizenship in 46 BC. One of the first Greek doctors to move to Rome was Asclepiades of Prus in Bithynia. Successful not only as a doctor but also as a teacher, Asclepiades, who found the Hippocratic system of medicine too passive, compiled about twenty books in which he expressed his preference for strict dietetics, as also for all kinds of physical therapy – for baths and gymnastics, active and passive movements, warm and cold remedies, sunbathing, etc. Asclepiades was a man of many talents; he also occupied himself with the healing properties of different kinds of wine – a practice which enhanced his popularity – and his special interest was in the study of mental illness.

The prestige of the Greek doctors in Rome quickly grew, so

much so that Emperor Augustus even elevated his personal doctor to the nobility. Fortunately the curb of scepticism was not long-lived. Interest in detailed anatomy had once more been aroused by the time Ruphos of Ephesus was practising in Rome in about the year A.D 100. He succeeded, among other things, in making the momentous discovery of the optic chiasma, a great step forward in the history of medicine; other aspects of his work were concerned with malignant tumours and the plague. He, too, was the author of a book on sphygmology.

Another Greek doctor, in whom the true Alexandrian-Hellenistic spirit of research lived on, and who became well known in Rome during the second century AD, was Soran, who was also from Ephesus. Since scepticism was still not completely conquered, he, too, had to make some excuse for his interest in anatomy, namely that 'An interest in anatomy might be useless, but would act as an adornment to the doctor of science.' So Soran, who was regarded as the great gynaecologist of ancient times, turned to the subject of his special interest, the female organs. He compiled a manual on the construction and functions of the female organs, including menstruation, conception, pregnancy, birth and the processes of reproduction. He also wrote an essay on human semen.

Soran's name is comparatively little-known; far greater is the fame of another doctor of Greek origin, who worked in Rome during the second century AD. His name was Galenus of Pergamum. He was destined to be the most famous doctor of classical antiquity after Hippocrates, though it is true to say that with him the creative period of classical Greek medicine came to an end.

10

*Claudius Galenus, the fashionable doctor
of imperial Rome. Galen, the most
important experimentalist of medical
history before the seventeenth century.
Galen's death brings to an end scientific,
anatomical and physiological investigation
for the time being.*

Claudius Galenus was born in
Pergamum in the summer of AD 129. Pergamum, home of Attalus
and capital of Mysia, was situated in Asia Minor not far from
the Aegean coast opposite the island of Lesbos. The city, which
once contained a famous library and shrine to Aesculapius, and
its name have been familiar to antiquarians since the beginning
of this century, when archaeologists excavated the immense altar
frieze on the castle mound. In a vividly naturalistic style, this
frieze depicted the battle between the gods and giants.

Socrates was not the only one to have his Xanthippe; in one
of his many books, Galen's youthful memories make this clear.
His father, Nikon, the architect, was a kind-hearted man, but his
mother was very different. She was a quarrelsome, obsessively
argumentative woman, always ill-tempered, ceaselessly abusive,
and so uncontrolled that she sometimes even bit the housemaids
during her outbreaks of violent passion.

Claudius Galenus inherited qualities from both parents. If
legend can be believed, it was a dream which decided his

93

father to make him become a doctor. Galen's early education was at the School of Philosophy in Pergamum; after his seventeenth year he also took lessons from the doctor, Satyros, who specialized in anatomy and is known to have written a manual on the subject.

His father, to whom he had been close, died when Galen was only twenty. Immediately afterwards Galen's years of wandering began. He visited Smyrna, then Corinth in Greece; but the city of Alexandria with its ancient and famous scientific atmosphere, drew him like a magnet. It was a city whose spirit, unlike that of Rome – the great capital of the world – led science and research to be pursued for their own sake. Thanks to this centuries-old tradition, it was in Galen's day still the kind of place where people were eagerly and actively concerned in solving the mystery of the human body. It was this spirit that still maintained its reputation as a citadel of anatomical studies, although nearly five hundred years had elapsed since Herophilus and Erasistratus had established its fame in this sphere. Galen had hardly arrived in that city on the Nile delta when this passion for research gripped him, that intoxicating joy in the discovery of life's secrets which was to remain with him for the rest of his life.

True, conditions in Alexandria were no longer as favourable as they had been in the time of the Ptolemies, whose era had ended in 30 BC with the death of Caesar's favourite, Cleopatra. Under the Roman aegis, dissection of human bodies was strictly forbidden. Galen therefore had to obtain his practical experience from the dissection of animals. This was the first reason for the many errors in his teaching; the conclusions he arrived at from his studies of the inner organs of animals such as pigs, goats and monkeys, he applied without hesitation to human beings.

During his thirtieth year, Galen gave up his wandering life and, with a certificate to prove he had passed his examinations, he returned to his native Pergamum to practise as a doctor. His luck was in. The summer festival was about to begin, but there was no doctor to attend the gladiatorial combats. Galen stepped into the breach and was so successful in treating the dreadful wounds that he continued to do so for several years, in addition to building up a growing private practice in the city. Four years after his return, however, he found Pergamum too limited for his rapidly expanding horizons.

In the second century AD what magnet was there to draw an ambitious young scientist? There could only be one answer: Rome. In AD 161, Galen set off for the imperial city. Although he may have found fame in his native Pergamum, in the great city of Rome he was one of many and at first no one noticed him. However, luck was again on his side. A well-known philosopher – a member of the Pergamumian colony in Rome – fell ill with malaria and, after several other doctors had already tried in vain to cure him, Galen succeeded where they had failed.

The young doctor's first cure was like a stone cast into a pool. The ripples spread and in no time at all his name was on everyone's lips, the number of his aristocratic patients grew and from then it was only a step to the court of Caesar.

Here, again, luck was with him. One of Caesar's chief administrators, whose wife he had cured of a female complaint, was an enthusiastic amateur student of anatomy. Galen immediately knew how to take advantage of his patron's hobby. Together they dissected the corpses of animals and everything that Galen observed he recorded. But again Galen made the mistake of applying slavishly to human conditions all that he saw in the animals' bodies.

By the time Galen had been in Rome four years, he had a brilliant practice as the favourite physician of many aristocratic patrons, and was commanding immense fees. Suddenly he felt drawn back to Pergamum, his birthplace. Was he tired of court life or were there other reasons why he left Rome? It is possible that Galen left Rome because of the virulent outbreak of smallpox which the returning Roman legionaries brought back from the Parthian wars and which claimed an immense number of victims. This, and many other considerations, such as the fact that he was by no means modest, indicate that Galen had inherited a streak of his mother's character. Certainly he did not, in his exalted position, measure up to his great predecessor, Hippocrates, who calmly stayed on in Athens during an equally serious epidemic.

However, Galen's stay in Pergamum was only brief; the 'philosopher emperor' Marcus Aurelius called him back to the capital and, by the end of AD 160, Galen was again in Rome. This time he was to remain there for thirty years during which period his life was filled with ceaseless activity: work as doctor to the imperial court, research, lectures, dissertations and discussions and last, but not least, tireless work as a writer – for Galen wrote more than thirty books.

Despite the fact that numerous areas of Galen's teachings were erroneous, he added many important observations and discoveries to the knowledge of anatomy. Many aspects of his essays on the construction and functions of the body in particular surpass much that had been written before his time. His research into the nervous system was particularly distinguished in that he discerned the difference between the nerves of the spinal cord and those in the cranium. He added to existing knowledge of the brain a series of significant new details, though it is true that he assumed a mistaken connection between the brain and the nasal cavity and believed that air reached the brain via the roof of the nose. He also remained firm in his conviction that the nervous system consisted of a network of pipes, possessing a direct connection with the ventricles of the brain, which he had already described with great care. He believed the ventricles of the brain were filled with *Pneuma* (vital spirit) and that every time they contracted in a pulsatory manner, this *pneuma* was forced down the nerve pipes.

Correct assumption is strangely mingled with confused conceptions of the work of the heart, the vascular system and the blood in the human body. Of really lasting significance was Galen's demonstration that arteries were filled with blood and not with air, as was believed by Aristotle and his successors. Admittedly this was a pardonable mistake – and one which even a great scholar such as Erasistratus shared – for, after death the arteries automatically become bloodless. Galen, on the other hand, taught that the arteries did not carry air but blood and that this arterial blood was charged with vital spirit while passing through the lungs. If the rather vague concept *spiritus vitalis* or 'vital spirit' is replaced by the word 'oxygen', then it is quite astonishing how close Galen came to the truth.

His views on the flow of humours in the body seem very fanciful. In the liver, he said, food was turned into blood. This manufactured blood was then carried to the vessels of the body where the ebb and flow of body juices was maintained by the pumping action of the heart. With unyielding obstinacy, Galen maintained in his teachings the ancient doctrine that the septum dividing the right side of the heart from the left contained porous areas and that blood seeped through these 'pores' in order to be carried further round the body. Heart and lungs, however, were connected by the trachea so that air could reach the (left) heart from the lungs, to cool and infuse the blood with vital spirit.

Doubtless Galen's chief contribution to medicine was his zealous promotion of anatomical and physiological knowledge. In his medical work he unreservedly acknowledged his debt to Hippocrates and felt called upon to continue the development of medical science begun by the old patriarch. Even in this conviction he did not suffer from modesty. In one of his verbose tracts containing both attacks on his colleagues and a fair measure of self-praise he wrote: 'I have never been as faulty in prognosis or therapy as many other highly reputable doctors. If, however, there is anyone who would like to be famous, not just for ingenious speeches but for deeds as well, then all he need do is to absorb without effort what I have spent a whole lifetime of eager research in discovering.'

Elsewhere Galen mentioned that the Emperor Marcus Aurelius

had said of him: 'We have only one doctor and he is a respectable one ...' and he added that the emperor had described him as the most distinguished doctor and philosopher, for he had tried many others before Galen and not only had they shown a grasping love of money, but they were quarrelsome, vain, envious and spiteful as well.

Unsuccessfully Galen tried to merge the theory of body humours or juices, which he had adopted from the work of Hippocrates and Aristotle, with a theory of organs and his own concept of *pneuma* and *pthisis*, taking from each of these whatever suited his train of thought at the time. From Aristotle he took the principle that nature never does anything fruitlessly.

In contrast to his great predecessor, Hippocrates, Galen believed that the cause of an illness was local in origin. He was one of the first to state that pus is a necessary accompaniment to the healing of a wound, and thus arrived at the 'praiseworthy pus' concept. He was incomparably more active in therapy than 'the father of medicine' had been; to him bleeding and purging were everyday remedies, nor was he sparing of medicines. Commensurate with the high esteem in which medical plants were held, his prescriptions were often compounded of a great many different ingredients which is why, to this day, such medicines are described as 'Galenic' preparations. Galen also paid great attention to hygiene; he, too, believed that prevention was better than cure.

Claudius Galenus died at the age of seventy. He had based his work as much on commonsense as experience, and his death brought to an end a strenuous and fruitful life. As pointed out by the medical historian, Erwin H. Ackerknecht, Galen was unquestionably the most important medical experimentalist, not only of his own time, but of all medical history before the seventeenth century.

Nevertheless, his sometimes flagrant mistakes had particularly serious consequences. Everyone who has tried to discover the secrets of the human body and the laws of medicine has been subject to error; it was so thousands of years ago and is still so today. The reason why Galen's misconceptions had such serious results for over a thousand years was that his death brought to an end all scientific, anatomical and physiological research. Therefore, what he had taught remained an inviolable precept, so much so that, during the Middle Ages, with its blind belief in authority – and even during the early part of modern times – it was nothing short of sacrilege to question Galen's teachings in any way.

I I

The status of doctors and medicine during the decline of the Roman Empire; comparatively high development of surgery. After the fall of Rome, medicine returns into the control of the priests; clerical doctors. Stagnation, paralysis and decay of medical science; the monks' belief in demons; the first hospitals are started in the cloisters.

When the philosopher emperor, Marcus Aurelius, died of the Antonine scourge, smallpox – in spite of the efforts of his personal physician Galen – a sad period began for imperial Rome. A life of idleness and luxury, immorality and corruption, despotism, extremely high taxation, and a decline in agriculture spread throughout the land. It is self-evident that these manifestations of dissolution also affected the doctors. Hardly anything remained of the high ideals embodied in the oath or the professional ethics originated by Hippocrates, the father of medicine; quack doctors and charlatans prospered, fashionable doctors became millionaires.

Even in Galen's day, the prospects of maintaining the standards of the profession were poor. Young doctors were not interested in acquiring knowledge, in practising the art of healing or of serving their fellow men; their sole aim was to transact the business as quickly as possible, and translate their medical skill into hard cash. It is thanks to Galen's angry complaints about the growing signs of decadence that we are particularly well informed of this state of affairs. He reported that when he wanted to teach his pupils about the construction of the human body and the function of its organs, they told him not to bore them with such absurd matters. Full of bitterness, he went on to say: 'The only difference between a robber and a doctor is that the former commits his crimes in the mountains and the latter commits them in Rome.'

As mentioned earlier, Rome's contribution to the development of medical science was slight. Nevertheless, it would be unjust to overlook what was accomplished, for example in the field of public health and hygiene which shows marked signs of the Etruscan influence. The ruins of palatial baths – found chiefly in Rome, but also in many other parts of the empire – still fill us with awe and astonishment. It should also be remembered that every Roman house was supplied with fresh water by means of a system of aqueducts, that water closets have been excavated and that, even during Rome's earliest days, the *cloaca maxima* drained the marshes around the hills and kept the city clean. The existence of sickness insurance and medical associations seems entirely modern.

Rome also contributed much to the status of the medical profession. Even in the days of Augustus, doctors were exempt from paying taxes and when, during Caesar's reign, there was a shortage of food and all foreigners – about eighty thousand – were forced to settle in the colonies, the doctors, the great majority of whom were foreigners, were exempt. Vespasian and Hadrian extended these privileges to include exemption from military service. At the beginning of the third century AD, Septimius Severus established a certificate of medical qualification.

However, it was by no means only foreigners, that is to say Greeks, who were practising in Rome; there were also pure-blooded Romans engaged in the art of healing. Best known of these was Aulus Cornelius Celsus, who lived during the regency of Emperor Tiberius and was a jack-of-all-trades. He was well versed in rhetoric, philosophy, politics, jurisprudence and the art of war, as well as that of healing. He also wrote a number of treatises, but all have been lost save the eight books *De re Medica*. These convey a clear picture of the position then occupied by medical science. Especially instructive are his comments on the art of surgery which show the comparatively high standard reached in Ancient Rome. Operations for hernia and goitre, removal of tonsils and cataract – even facial operations – are described in minute detail. Moreover, anyone visiting the excavations at Pompeii, the town near Naples which was buried under lava and ashes after the eruption of Vesuvius on 24 August 79 AD, can judge for himself the high standard of surgery which existed. The route to the ruins runs past a small museum where numerous surgical instruments, found during the excavations, are on display. In many ways they resemble those in use today.

Finally, it should be remembered that it was Roman farmers and architects who first voiced the suspicion that malaria, which was especially prevalent in Latium (the present-day Campagna) was caused by a tiny creature originating in the marshes. The construction of dwellings was adapted in an attempt to counter this threat, but none of the measures taken were able to stem the attacks of 'marsh fever'.

A particularly devastating malarial epidemic spread through the Roman Empire during the third century AD. This epidemic doubtless reinforced the other causes already mentioned which contributed to the decline and fall of the Roman Empire. Almost the entire ruling civilized stratum of society was swept away by malaria at that time. The native Romans were not as immune to malaria as were their slaves who had originated in malarial lands, and consequently the latter were gradually able to achieve an ascendancy over the pure-blooded Romans.

Meanwhile, the most important historical revolution of all time loomed on the horizon. Christianity had made immense advances and, although there were still occasional persecutions, the martyrdom and loss of believers seemed only to strengthen the religious community. Already membership of the Christian faith had spread into the highest circles; Diocletian's wife Prisca and his daughter, Valeria, openly sympathized with the new faith. It was through Constantine, who regarded the sun god as his protective deity, that freedom of faith was proclaimed by an official edict in Milan during the year AD 313. He was also the instigator of the division of the Roman Empire when, seventeen years later, he founded a second Rome, Byzantium, on the Bosphorus. On the pillar of Constantine, he is represented as the sun god surrounded by a brilliant aureole, holding the earthly globe in his hand and, surmounting the globe, stands the cross – two supposedly opposing faiths had been merged . . .

The decay of the Roman Empire was accelerated when, with the invasion of the Goths, Huns and Vandals, the people began to migrate. In AD 410 Rome was taken by the barbarians, and during the last quarter of the fifth century the western half of the Roman Empire disappeared; Byzantium, or Constantinople, was now the capital of the empire.

Scientific progress could not be expected during such chaotic times. It is true that one or two outstanding doctors kept alive the medical tradition; but they were merely healers of the sick, and in no way involved in medical research. Also, when Christianity became the ruling power, medical science did not have an easy time. This was because everything that had any connection with science, whether it was in philosophy, natural science or medicine, seemed to the Christians to hark back to 'heathendom', and to savour of the devil. The founder of the Cistercian Order was even of the opinion that to buy medicine, consult a doctor or swallow any kind of medical preparation was irreconcilable with the Christian religion.

Under such conditions, it is not surprising that the medical profession seems to have been wholly neglected. However, since there are always some sick people who are grateful for any advice in their adversity, they began to turn to the clergy for help. The wheel had come full circle; medical science again fell into the hands of the priests and the results were not long in appearing. The old superstition was revived that sickness was a punishment from heaven for sins committed; the remedies of the Church – constant prayer and the laying on of hands – replaced medical skill. Once more the conjuring up of spirits, the black arts and a belief in magic, proliferated. It seems almost incredible that a person as eminent as Aurelius Augustinus, the most prominent father of the Western Church during the fifth century, could refer to the high rate of infant mortality in such terms as: 'the illnesses of Christians are called forth by demons who chiefly torment freshly baptized, yes, even innocent, new-born children'.

In view of such attitudes, it is hardly surprising that, at that time, there was no thought of a rational art of healing or of its development. The stagnation, paralysis and decay of every scientific activity set in. Productive research ceased, many of the advances made in anatomy, physiology and medicine were forgotten; instead of depending upon science, people relied on clerical superstition. Nevertheless, anyone studying medical history will appreciate the efforts of those young Christian clerics who worked so hard in the monasteries to preserve and record the little that survived the collapse of classical antiquity and who carried it forward into the Middle Ages.

In the realm of ethics, however, progress is unmistakable. The medical instruction that incurable diseases should not be treated, which is met in so many ancient civilizations and even in Hippocrates' teachings, was replaced by the introduction of the Christian duty of charity even towards hopeless cases. Another true advance was the establishment of sick-wings in many monasteries and even proper hospitals, although the medicine taught in monastery schools inevitably acquired a clerical character. Herb gardens sprang up here and there when it was realized that patients needed help other than prayers or the laying on of hands; and when clerical doctors began to lose their mistrust of rational medicine, they took pains to combine the Christian doctrine of faith with ancient wisdom.

It is worth noting that, during the Middle Ages, women were also active in healing. The most well-known of these is Hildegard von Bingen who was abbess of the Rupertsberg convent during the twelfth century. With her, too, a naturalistic conception of illness was strangely interwoven with an early Christian belief in devils. She received revelations in visions which commanded: 'Write down what you see and hear.' True to these commands, during the course of eight years she dictated to two monks a book about natural history and another on medicine. Very sensibly recognizing a basic need, she organized her nuns to provide an outstanding health service. In a unique compromise she combined the requirements of a rational concept of illness with Christian superstition. It was vitally necessary, she maintained, to strengthen the sick body so that it could better withstand the attacks of the devil and his confederates.

The scope of psychotherapy in medieval medical thinking is proved by, among other things, the method of healing which involved the laying on of hands. According to a popular belief, anointed kings possessed the power to cure diseases by laying their consecrated royal hands on the head or nape of the neck of the sick person. Chlodwig I, King of the Franks, made use of this ceremony as early as the end of the fifth century; in England the practice was introduced during the eleventh century under Edward the Confessor, particularly for use in cases of scrofula. This procedure goes back to the gospel of St Mark where it says: 'They shall lay hands on the sick, and they shall recover.' During the ceremony, in which as many as a thousand or even fifteen hundred people might be treated at one session, the king would lay his hands on the head or nape of the person who was sick, uttering the words: 'I touch you, God heals you.'

Monastic and clerical medicine came to an end during the twelfth century after the Synod of Clermont. Monks were then forbidden to pursue any healing activities because these conflicted too much with the real purpose of monasticism – unworldly piety.

12

After a detour to Arabia, classical medicine returns to the West, retranslated by Constantine the African, from Arabic back into Latin. The Arabic doctors Al Rhazi and Avicenna. The medical school of Salerno was the seed from which the medical faculties of the future were to spring.

After a strangely tortuous detour, the medical science of classical antiquity which had been half lost or forgotten, returned to the West during the Middle Ages. In 570 Mohammed was born in Mecca. He hated the idolatry and fetishism of the Arabs and preached to his countrymen the doctrine of one almighty and omniscient God. Apart from his inner vocation, contact with Christians living in Arabia – as a businessman Mohammed had to make many journeys – may have been one of the causes for his monotheistic ideas.

When he was sixty years old, he experienced the triumph of his teaching in Arabia, although the spread of the new religion throughout the Mediterranean under the first caliphs only took place after his death. Syria, Palestine, Babylon, Persia, Egypt, North Africa, Spain and large parts of India were brought under its sway, and one century after the prophet's death, the Arabian kingdom stretched from the Indus to the Pyrennees.

The wild hordes, who began by spreading the teaching of Allah and his prophet by fire and sword, settled and became a com-

munity made up of different races and peoples united by a belief
in the Koran and – since any translation was forbidden – by the
Arabic language. A new civilization flourished which was to
hold its own for more than five hundred years. Existing knowledge that had been found was absorbed and given new form;
with almost youthful ardour people learnt all they could from
foreign artists and scientists. At first Damascus in Syria was the
capital of this vast empire, then ancient Baghdad took its place.
Magnificent buildings rose up from the ground; schools, academies and libraries are evidence of the new masters' thirst for
knowledge.

Alexandria was still a focal point of the sciences and especially
of medicine. The famous library there, the biggest in antiquity,
with its seven hundred thousand book rolls, had perished in the
flames long ago during 48 and 47 BC, when Caesar's soldiers had
fought the Egyptians in Alexandria.

Nevertheless, there were still accounts of the ancient sciences –
though widely distributed – in numerous books, and the Arab
conquerors were avid to lay hands on them. Diplomatic missions
searched everywhere for such books; in peace treaties one of the
conditions required the handing over of such works. So a great
Moslem library grew up in Baghdad which was not inferior to
its Alexandrian predecessor. The Arabs soon learned that the
treatments and prescriptions worked out by Greek doctors were
more effective than the traditional Arabic mumbo jumbo, so
they went to work eagerly to translate those of the old books
which had been preserved.

One of these translation centres grew up in Gondeshapur
(Persia) where the schools of the Nestorian or Chaldean Christians
were active in transmitting Greek scientific knowledge. Because
of its location, the discovery of works by ancient authors, particularly from the Orient, resulted in a faithful synthesis of
oriental and Greek medical skills. However, it would be wrong
to assume that Arabic medicine was merely an offshoot from the
Greek. On the contrary, Arab specialists – especially eye-doctors

– enjoyed a high reputation. The development of surgery, it is true, was hindered because of the Moslem fear of shedding blood and so the branding iron had to replace the scalpel.

Medical chemistry, on the other hand, experienced a considerable revival under the Arabs; the word 'alcohol', for example, is of pure Arabic origin. It was also because of this interest in human chemistry that the examination of urine played such a commanding role in diagnostics. During the following centuries this significance was to increase; and there is hardly a picture of a medieval doctor who is not busy studying a sample of urine. The study of pharmacology reached such proportions that it became necessary, at the beginning of the eighth century, to separate for the first time the profession of doctor from that of chemist. Magnificent hospitals were built, the most famous of them in Damascus and Cairo, which were also used for the training of young doctors. Then an indigenous Arabic medical literature began to evolve; two outstanding doctors – Al Rhazi and Avicenna – being especially concerned in its creation. Al Rhazi, whose real name was, in fact, Abu Bekr Mohammed Ibn Zakkariya, came from Persian Khorasan which had only been conquered by the Caliphs around the middle of the seventh century. He was born in the year 865 and can be regarded as an Arabic intellectual all-rounder. However his chief interest was not, at first, in medicine. He studied philosophy, mathematics, physics, astronomy and music and it was only a chance meeting which led him towards medical science. Frequent visits to a hospital, as well as detailed discussions with a great friend of his, an old chemist who worked at the hospital, caused Al Rhazi's interest in medicine to grow until finally he spent all his time studying medical science. Moreover he showed such a talent for it that he soon became a well-known doctor and was appointed head of the hospital.

Al Rhazi collected a great many pupils and, from time to time, he was also summoned to the court at Baghdad. He was an extraordinarily prolific writer of medico-literary works and is said to have written more than a hundred books – some say more than two hundred. His best-known work, a manual on medicine which he dedicated to the king of Khorasan, also had a far-reaching effect on Western healing. His monographs on smallpox, measles and children's diseases also prove how extraordinarily observant he was. His longest work, however, is the vast encyclopaedia, *El Hawl*, which collects together all Greek, Arabic and Indian medical knowledge and experience, and which relies on the description of typical case histories.

Just over a century after Al Rhazi, another doctor became famous. He was called Avicenna. His real name, Abu Ali Husain ibn Abdullah ibn Siba, was no less impressive than that of his predecessor. Avicenna, too, was a Persian and he was born in AD 980, in the neighbourhood of Bukhara. Like Al Rhazi, he had already developed into an intellectual all-rounder in his youth and was equally at home in mathematics, physics, philosophy, dialectics, jurisprudence, theology and metaphysics.

This infant prodigy began to study medicine when he was sixteen years old; at eighteen he was already a well-known doctor who was summoned to the court, and at twenty-one he compiled an encyclopaedia of sciences containing a twenty-volume commentary. Besides studying, writing, teaching and practising as a doctor in many far-flung localities whose names are known to us today as the places of origin of valuable carpets, he was appointed minister of State. Constitutionally, however, he was unable to bear such a multifarious burden indefinitely and he died, in 1037, at the age of fifty-seven. In his five-part *Canon* of Greek-Arabic medical sciences, which is still regarded as the catechism of healing in the Middle East, Avicenna succeeded in doing what Galen had tried in vain to accomplish: to establish a complete system of medical science.

In the east of the vast Arab empire, therefore, where the Caliphs ruled with incomparably more tolerance and liberality than the Christian Church did in her domains, the ancient classical medicine, permeated with Arabic science, had quickly blossomed.

In the West, on the other hand, the lost knowledge of the old masters still lay dormant; here it was not until the turn of the tenth century that a doctor, Constantine of Africa, reawakened interest in the old sciences. He was a man who had travelled widely; ranging, for nearly four decades, over Mesopotamia, India, Ethiopia and Egypt in order to study the medicine of the ancient civilizations in their places of origin. In the monastery of Monte Cassino he at last found a resting place, and in that peaceful monastery he created the work that has made him immortal: he re-translated the ancient medical classics from the Arabic back into Latin.

In this way Greek medical science returned to the West by a strange detour; by way of the new Rome, or Constantinople, it had reached Syria and Persia to become Arabic knowledge, and now it found its way back to Italy through the translations of the African, Constantine. At once the old science began to put out fresh shoots from its new graft, and the oldest medical school in the West, the one in Salerno, became the first famous centre of medicine of the Middle Ages.

Originating in a pilgrim hospital attached to a Benedictine monastery, the Salernian school again freed medicine from the control of the priests. It had not been founded by the clergy but by laymen and places were available for both men and women of all nationalities, speaking many languages, to undergo medical training. Soon its fame as a first-class training hospital spread; the medical school of Salerno was already mentioned in Hartmann von Aue's masterpiece *Der Arme Heinrich* (Poor Henry) written about AD 1200. In this a doctor from Salerno tells Henry, who is suffering from leprosy, that his only hope is to obtain the heart's blood of a pure maiden who is willing to die for him.

The outstanding and balanced syllabus of Salerno was shown to be so successful that it was later adopted by the great universities. A number of publications brought out by the school of Salerno illustrate the high standard of the combination of Greek and Arabic classical medicine; particularly able essays describe the dysenteric intestinal diseases and the diseases of the urinary passages. The treatment of endemic goitre with marine products containing iodine, still in use today, was well known then; for skin diseases ointments containing mercury were used. In the realms of surgery, instructions concerning intestinal sutures are particularly astonishing. If it is remembered how many centuries were to pass before women were again allowed to attend medical lectures at the universities in modern times, it must be conceded that the school of Salerno was remarkably broad-minded in this respect alone. True, what they achieved in surgery for example, was judged in an extremely disparaging way. Nevertheless a Salernian woman doctor published a book about female diseases and baby care, and she was also well-versed in cosmetics for she recommended a decoction made of elderberry, broom, egg-yolks and saffron for giving a golden sheen to the hair.

The work of a medical scholar at the academy of Salerno represents a unique phenomenon. In this work, which was written around AD 1140, professional cunning and medical ethics intermingle in a most amusing manner. The book advises a doctor, as soon as he is called out on a case, to find out from the messenger as much as he can about the past history and present condition of his client so that the latter and his immediate circle will be filled with astonishment by the physician's knowledge. Doctors apparently knew quite a lot about the connection between the circulation and the emotions for he goes on to say: 'Feel his pulse, but remember, while doing so, that it may well be affected by your presence or, if your patient should be a skinflint, by the thought of your fee ...' His advice not to be hasty with diagnosis or prognosis demonstrates great worldly wisdom for, 'the friends or family will be grateful for a verdict upon which they have had to wait for a time'. Equally prudent seems the recommendation that the doctor should tell the patient that with God's help he will cure him, while, at the same time telling relatives that the case is a serious one. This practice is certainly still widespread.

At times the presence of the patient's female relatives must have been a great temptation to doctors for, like every other code of professional ethics, the Salernian one says: 'Beware of casting acquisitive eyes on a man's maidservant, or daughter, or his wife...'

A great service rendered by the medical school in Salerno was the reintroduction of a kind of medical licence – the first since Septimius Severus. Around the middle of the twelfth century, Roger II, King of Sicily, Calabria and Apulia, enacted a statute according to which no one was allowed to practise medicine without a certificate of qualification. This law was also a prelude to the systematic sanitary regulations introduced about a century later by Emperor Frederick II of Hohenstaufen.

The medical school in Salerno was elevated to the rank of a public college in 1220 and flourished until well into the thirteenth century. It enjoyed such a reputation that a doctor who could say he had received his professional training there was universally trusted. When, later, other bigger establishments came into being, Salerno gradually diminished in importance. This does not, however, alter the fact that the college of Salerno was the seed from which the medical faculties in the great universities of later times were to spring.

13

Medicine returns to the control of the priests; Arnold of Villanova and Pietro d'Abano. After the establishment of the Inquisition independent research and ideas become dangerous. Roger Bacon, a light in the darkness. The Order of the Holy Ghost founded the first poorhouses, hospitals and orphanages.

As mentioned in the previous chapter, Emperor Frederick II of Hohenstaufen enacted sanitary regulations and introduced doctor's licences during the 1230s. Prior to this, in 1225, he founded the University of Naples. He also initiated a nine-year medical course which ended with a state examination; he introduced the professional establishment of doctors, rules governing fees, pharmaceutical regulations and public instructions regarding hygiene. This emperor's work alone refutes the frequently made charge that during the Middle Ages medical science lay dormant.

The University of Naples was to become a dangerous rival to the Salerno college and, as universities had already been established in other places, the importance of the college began to wane. The oldest of these universities was that of Paris, founded in 1110. Next came Bologna in 1113, Oxford in 1167 and Montpellier in 1181. During the thirteenth century universities were established in Messina and Padua; during the fourteenth century in Prague, Vienna, Heidelberg, Cologne and Erfurt.

The everlasting circle now brought medicine back into the hands of the priests, for the professors teaching medical science at the universities were ecclesiastics and in some places even had to take vows of celibacy. For the rest, medicine had to adapt itself to the Church's conception of the world and wherever the Pope acted as patron to a university, medical science became the veritable handmaid of theology. Nevertheless, what was really new was that at different places in Europe there existed establishments for a systematic medical training; particularly at the universities of Montpellier, Bologna and Padua, which produced doctors whose names have come down to us through the centuries.

The only medical man ever to acquire papal dignity was Petrus Hispanicus, who became Pope Peter Johannes XXI. He obtained his medical qualifications at the University of Montpellier; the same university also produced Arnold of Villanova, a native of Portugal, who practised medicine during the second half of the thirteenth century. He, like the other doctors of his time, can count as belonging to the scholastic period of medicine. This did not produce any original medical ideas of its own, but was more concerned, as a result of an unshakeable belief in authority, to present the reinstated Greek teaching without any addition of personal experience; to analyse, comment and explain. Nevertheless, practical medicine owes thanks to Arnold in one important respect: he was the first to prepare tinctures of vegetable matter based on alcohol and he also invented brandy which he called *aqua vitae* or water of life.

Characteristic of the high repute which educated doctors enjoyed at that time is that Villanova, like a number of his colleagues, was entrusted with important diplomatic missions. But the esteem in which he was held was not able to prevent him from coming into conflict with the Church. This conflict was all the more pronounced as he did not restrict himself to medical studies, but also debated philosophical and theological matters. The Inquisition prosecuted him and he would doubtless have been burnt, together with his writings, if he had not been the personal friend and protégé of Pope Boniface VIII.

Only a short time after Arnold of Villanova, a doctor who had studied medicine and philosophy in Padua and who was probably acquainted with Dante caused a stir. His name was Pietro d'Abano. It is unlikely that Pietro's professional activities were basically different from those of his colleague, Arnold of Villanova. As a result of the constant translation, retranslation and copying of the old texts, a number of obscurities, inconsistencies and often even contradictions had come into being. The scholarly doctors therefore regarded it as their task to rearrange the surviving ancient texts into logical order according to the dialectical ways demonstrated by Aristotle and the Arabs and to fit them all into a system.

In doing so, Pietro evidently, however, developed original ideas; and this at a time when independent thought was just as forbidden as the declaration of personal opinions was mortally dangerous. As a result he, too, ended up in the hands of the Inquisition, accused of magic and necromancy. He was only acquitted after protracted and hair-splitting legal proceedings.

In such circumstances it is not surprising that original research – and original thought in general – appeared to have died, though there were certainly men at that time who might have been capable of it. As things were, however, they preferred to restrict themselves to the study of the ancient texts sanctioned by the Church. This is why it is often said that during the Middle Ages medicine was less concerned with the sick-bed or the laboratory than with the library.

It follows also that no real progress – especially in anatomical studies – was achieved. Even occasional post-mortems, undertaken to solve crimes, for example, had as little impact on this state of affairs as the decree of Emperor Frederick II of Hohenstaufen, which permitted the dissection of a human body every five years!

What Galen had taught was sacrosanct to such an extent that people simply could not or would not see anything different.

The branch of medicine which was in the worst plight during the Middle Ages was surgery. The Synod of Tours, which sat in AD 1163, had announced dogmatically: '*Ecclesia abhorret a sanguine*' (i.e. the Church abhors any form of bloodshed). It has already been mentioned that in those days all doctors were priests; therefore they could not contravene the commands of the Church. Thus surgery slipped out of the hands of the doctors and became the craft of all kinds of shadowy practitioners such as the castrator, the travelling quack, the hangman and the barber.

Even here there were honourable exceptions. One of these was the doctor, Guy de Chauliac, who was of French farming stock and who studied medicine and theology in Montpellier. He rose to become the domestic chaplain and personal physician to several of the popes. In worthy contrast to the lowly position occupied by surgery at that time, Guy de Chauliac was an excellent surgeon who effected a decisive improvement in operations for stones and for cataracts. He also compiled a work, *Chirurgia Magna*, which described a large number of innovations, many of which are still in use today. Guy de Chauliac was the originator of the procedure – still practised today – by means of which extension bandages and weights are applied in cases of bone fracture, in order to prevent malformities during healing, by stretching the limb in a longitudinal direction.

Surgeons of the calibre of Guy de Chauliac were, however, the exception in those days; anatomy and, as a logical result, also surgery, were the orphans of medieval medicine. Nevertheless, during that period of the Middle Ages there were some spirits who were far in advance of their time and, like distant flashes of lightning, announced the impending rise of an entirely new era in human history. Chief among these can be counted the thirteenth century English scholar, Roger Bacon, whose brilliant light illumined the darkness of his times. Bacon, who has justly been described as 'the first martyr in the cause of true research', was at one and the same time doctor, philosopher, natural scientist, mathematician and physicist. He had studied in Oxford, then in Paris, and while the learned men of his time were racking their brains over the scholarly subtleties of Aristotelian philosophy, while theological doctrines and dogmas were holding back all free research, and while life in the monasteries declined into idleness, gluttony and lewdness, the young Bacon was irresistibly drawn towards natural science and experimental research. The thoughtless repetition of the principles propounded by the Greek ancients was an abomination to him; the study of nature, of life, human and animal, was dear to his heart. His craving for knowledge was so great that, in order to find out about the internal organs of living creatures, he even dissected human and animal corpses. Bacon said that if it lay in his power, he would have all Aristotle's books burnt. He thought studying them was but time lost, and they only served to spread error and ignorance. Book learning had turned the heads of youth for long enough, he felt, and kept them from the true, direct study of nature. He begged people to lay aside the book of the ancients and turn to a study of the great book of nature which lay open to every one.

How successful Roger Bacon was in pursuing this study is best shown by the fact that he was thoroughly familiar with the human brain and every detail of the eye, that he knew about light-refraction by the lens, had seen the optic chiasma, was the first person to invent a pair of spectacles for presbyopic sight and very probably also anticipated the construction of the telescope so that Galileo Galilei was later able to continue his researches.

His far-reaching insight into the forces of nature is further shown by his prophecy that one day people would construct mechanically propelled boats 'so that they shall be able to drive across the seas at a speed unequalled by no matter how great a number of oarsmen ... it is possible to build a machine with big wings inside which a man may sit and fly through the air at a great speed like a bird. It will be possible to travel fast in a cart without horses or oxen. A small instrument will be able to lift great weights and loads.' All these prophecies are instantly reminiscent of a greater man who lived centuries later: Leonardo da Vinci.

As already mentioned earlier, it was in the highest degree dangerous to develop, or even utter, independent ideas. So Roger Bacon could not escape the Dominicans who, on orders from the Inquisition, were hot on the scent in search of heretics. It was only a short time previously that the great spiritual leader, Thomas Aquinas, *doctor comunis* and *doctor angelicus,* is said to have uttered the words which can probably only be understood in the context of those times: 'Heretics deserve not only to be excommunicated from the congregation of the Church, but to be separated from the world by death . . .'

These words would certainly have been applied to Roger Bacon if he had not had influential friends among the princes of the Church; so he was only buried alive for many years in a prison. Only a few years before his death, in the tomb-like atmosphere of his confinement, he wrote the work: *Methods of Preventing the Appearance of Senility* which represents a guide to a healthy and hygienic regimen. When, after a new pope had ascended St Peter's throne, he was at last released from the tomb of his prison, he was a tired, broken old man with only two more years ahead before he died at the age of eighty.

His legacy, however, was to prove immortal. He believed that a complete perception of the technical possibilities and the arts could only be achieved by experimental methods and that only by these methods could magic and enchantment be perceived to be nonsense, but this thought of his was, it is true, only given full recognition centuries later.

At the time when they were written, stubborn authoritarianism, narrow-minded dogmatism and scholarly sophistry were still the ruling principles.

Much more pleasant than the fate of the few bold spirits who, scorning all persecution, hurried far in advance of their times, is a description of hospitals during the Middle Ages.

There are many hospitals today which still bear the name, Hospital of the Holy Ghost. The title derives from the medieval Order of the Holy Ghost which, during the second half of the thirteenth century, had under its control more than a thousand subsidiary establishments. Among its many activities, this order became the originator of the present-day poor-houses, hospitals and orphanages.

During the crusades, which set out to conquer the Holy Land from the end of the eleventh century to the end of the thirteenth century, great numbers of sick, infirm and indigent people streamed back from Palestine. As a result towns in Europe were threatened by a flood of epidemics. This was the time when the great nursing orders were founded: the Order of the Knights of the Hospital of St John (or Hospitallers) in 1099; the Order of the Knights of the Temple (or Templars) and the Order of Lazarus (which devoted itself especially to the care of lepers) at the beginning of the twelfth century; and, at the end of the twelfth century, the Order of Teutonic Knights and the Order of the Holy Ghost. Founded by a Spanish nobleman, the Order of the Holy Ghost was sanctioned by Pope Innocent III.

On the initiative of the Order of the Holy Ghost, it became common practice for a chest with a hinged lid to be placed outside hospital doors, in which mothers could anonymously leave their babies. The order then took over all further care of the foundling. Holy Ghost hospitals, which looked after not just the sick but also the orphans, the poor, the cripples, the senile, the homeless and outcast, the disabled and mutilated, were established in many places, including Halberstadt, Eisenach, Erfurt, Stendal, Stettin, Königsberg, Regensburg, Memmingen, Landshut, Munich, Wasserburg am Inn, Fulda, Worms, Frankfurt and Pforzheim.

Quite apart from the Knights of the Cross, crusaders and their following, the Hospitallers also looked after the vast number of patients who found their way into the hospitals during epidemics great and small. Such epidemics were no rarity during the Middle Ages, as will be described in greater detail in the following chapter. An idea of the amount of work involved for the Hospitallers can be derived from the fact that, in the cemetery attached to the hospital of Dijon in France, more than ten thousand people who had died of the plague were buried during one year.

Just as, during the thirteenth century, one or two enlightened people anticipated the impending gigantic cultural revolution, so the coming change was also becoming gradually more noticeable in medicine as well. Henri de Mondeville (1268–1314), personal physician to King Philip the Fair of France, risked making the almost heretical statement: 'God had not quite exhausted his creative resources when he created Galen.' Rather, he urged his professional colleagues to a more diligent study of anatomy and, not long afterwards, true medical histories, based on observation, appeared at the big medical faculties once more. Ever more plainly the coming rebirth of the human spirit, known as the Renaissance, began to loom over the horizon; the end of the Middle Ages and the start of modern times was drawing near.

However, we cannot begin to describe this incisive change in history before mentioning a phenomenon which is regarded by some historians as the boundary between the beginning and end of the Middle Ages. This phenomenon was the great series of epidemics, particularly the plague.

14

*The great epidemics of the Middle Ages.
The Justinian plague of the sixth and the
Black Death of the fourteenth
century. Decline of morals, the beginning of
measures to promote public hygiene.
Leprosy and the English sweating sickness.
Mass frenzy and mass hysteria. The
flagellants and dancing mania. The children's
crusades.*

The period known as the Middle Ages lies between two great deadly epidemics: the Justinian plague, which raged in the sixth century during the reign of the Eastern Roman emperor Justinian, and the Black Death, which swept away a quarter of the population of Europe during the fourteenth century.

The epidemic which was named after Emperor Justinian is the first in history which can be described with certainty as being a plague epidemic. Even though the Ancient Mesopotamians had already connected the appearance of plague with the mass death of rats (see page 29), most of the epidemics described as 'plague' did not involve genuine cases of plague as we nowadays define the word. For example, recent research indicates that the Attic plague, the epidemic which Homer tells us raged in the Greek camp during the siege of Troy and ended the golden age of Athens, besides killing off Pericles, was not, in fact, plague.

Neither was the so-called Antonine plague, which the Roman legionaries brought back to Italy during the second century AD and which caused Marcus Aurelius' death. These were not genuine epidemics of plague, but epidemics of smallpox or typhus.

However, the Justinian plague which, during the year AD 542, killed ten thousand people in Constantinople alone, is the first epidemic in history which can be described with absolute certainty as being a mass epidemic of true bubonic plague. The description of its symptoms in contemporary accounts is unmistakable. The characteristic plague sore (bubo) in the groin and armpit is exactly as described; and it was known that its sloughing announced the patient's imminent death. The brilliant Greek historian Procopius, described the cruel course of the plague extremely vividly: 'No island', wrote Emperor Justinian's intimate, 'was so secluded, no cave or mountain peak so inaccessible, but the plague everywhere exacted its victims. No age was spared, no palace, no hut. People collapsed in the streets as if struck by lightning. They sank para-lysed to the ground before the altars. The streets became depopu-lated and filled with the stench of the corpses which littered the ground. Civil life had ceased; the only people left in the squares were the corpse-bearers... The plague weakened the influence of morals; those people who were not ill, abandoned themselves to the unbridled enjoyment of worldly pleasures and one was forced to believe that the disease had spared only the most de-praved specimens of humanity.'

Having died down, the plague only flamed up again in isolated cases here or there, but its virulence seemed broken. It only reawoke eight hundred years later – but this time with such force that in four months it wiped out forty-two million people. In Europe alone twenty-five million people died. The plague began in 1347 during a dry summer and travelled with terrifying speed westwards across India and south-west Russia. It is still possible to determine the place where it took off for Europe; this was the seaport then called Caffa, now known as Feodosiya, on the south-eastern tip of the Crimea in the Black Sea, and which served the city republics of Genoa and Venice as a base for their overseas commerce and as a port for the trans-shipment of merchandise for their trade with the Far East. When the Tartars, lured to Caffa by the warehouses belonging to the rich city republics, encircled and besieged the town, the Christian defenders were in a sore plight. They were on the point of surrendering when plague broke out in the Tartar camps. The besiegers died in their thousands and there was nothing left for the rest of the host but to flee back to the steppes from whence they had come.

Meanwhile, the jubilations of the besieged Christians at this unexpected change in their fortunes turned out to be premature. Before they moved off, the Tartars used their siege machines to catapult into the town a number of plague corpses. They achieved their object in full measure. The plague spread among the Italians with terrifying speed. Full of horror, the Christians embarked for home in their galleys, but most of the sailors died of plague before they ever reached Italy.

According to some reports, only ten out of a thousand refugees reached their home ports; and when they landed, the plague came with them. In no time it had travelled throughout Italy. It reached France on a ship which put in at Marseilles. Four-fifths of the inhabitants of this flourishing seaport fell prey to the disease. There was no route by water or overland which did not serve to spread the plague at lightning speed. It was not long before the epidemic was rife from the Far East to the North Sea, from Sicily to Greenland. Here, on the 'green island', death was so widespread, that the discovery of America, which had been made by the Norsemen one-and-a-half centuries before Columbus, was completely forgotten; so the man from Genoa was able to discover the New World again in 1492 (see also page 59).

The people believed that the end of the world had come. The disregard of all human morality was even more shocking than during the Justinian plague. Giovanni Boccaccio reported that, in the flourishing and populated city of Florence alone, a hundred thousand people died of the plague in a few months. He also described in detail the total destruction of morality in his introduction to the Decameron.

Medical science was powerless. Doctors who did not flee, convinced of the uselessness of their efforts, carried out their work dressed in fantastic protective clothing, which covered the face and was equipped with a beak-like container over the nose. This was filled with powerful aromatics intended to protect the doctor from the pestilential vapour; for in all contemporary reports the dreadful, unbearable stench of the plague sufferers and corpses is emphasized. From that day to this, the phrase 'pestilential smell' has remained in general use. Clothes were soaked in essences of amber, cinnamon, cloves, mace, attar of roses, camphor and saffron in order to keep away the plague stench; blazing fires were lit in the public squares; containers were set out filled with milk and freshly baked bread in order to bind the plague stench; some people even took a goat into their homes in order to superimpose the smell of goat over the stench of plague.

The plague-stricken themselves were purged, bled, sprinkled with aromatics, strengthened with theriaca, an ancient medicine composed of seventy ingredients which Andromachus of Crete, the personal physician of the Emperor Nero had discovered; the buboes were treated with poultices, thermo-cautery and knives; all was in vain. The belief that gluttony, drunkenness, overexcitement and anger encouraged the plague is thoroughly modern as is the conviction that to keep a balanced outlook would help one to escape the contagion.

When everything had been proved useless, and deaths from the plague assumed ever greater proportions, Pope Clement VI issued the well-meant proclamation calling for a pilgrimage to Rome for Easter 1348 in order to conquer the plague by the power of faith. The opposite was achieved. The plague raged worse than ever among the 1,200,000 people gathered together in Rome. If contemporary accounts can be believed, not even a tenth of the pilgrims was spared. To be sure the Pope had preferred not to take part in the pilgrimage himself but had stayed behind in Avignon, where he had shut himself up in one of the innermost rooms of his palace. He was, therefore, one of the survivors.

The people, turned half-mad by the horrors surrounding them, concocted the most fantastic ideas about the origin of the great death. Sometimes the stars were the cause, sometimes man's sinfulness until, in the end, they hit on the idea that the Jews were the malefactors. It was declared, in all seriousness, that they had poisoned the wells in order to exterminate Christianity from the face of the earth. When some wretched and persecuted individuals accused themselves of the most absurd deeds under torture, an unrestrained persecution of the Jews began to sweep through Europe. Entire Jewish communities were wiped out; in some places the Jews were simply driven into their synagogues which were then set on fire.

However, the plague did not produce exclusively negative consequences. It was soon noticed that uncleanliness, dirt and putrefaction helped to spread the plague and so strict regulations controlling hygiene were introduced into the cities. For the first time the authorities began to concern themselves with cleaning the streets; garbage, animal corpses and offal were no longer allowed to be thrown into the streets; they now had to be cleared away. Sick people, or those only suspected of suffering from plague, were kept strictly isolated; the bodies were removed at night and the possessions of the dead destroyed. Often the very houses in which the plague had been especially fierce were burnt.

It was also thanks to the plague that the so-called 'quarantines' were introduced. As people found that the epidemic was constantly being reintroduced via the waterways, the great Italian seaports were the first to accommodate foreigners, arriving by ship, in strictly guarded barracks outside the town, before allowing them to enter. Here they had to stay for forty days (*quaranta giorni*) before being allowed freedom of movement. So, as a result of the great plague, regulations governing public health came into being; the control of food in the markets had already preceded these.

The Black Death vanished as suddenly as it had come; but even though it had died down, this by no means meant the end of the plague in Europe. There were bad plague years even during the Renaissance which claimed, among others, a number of the most famous Italian painters as victims. Titian, aged ninety-nine was struck down by it while finishing his enormous picture, *The Mourning for Christ;* other victims were Ghirlandaio, Giorgione and Perugino. Various different countries were visited by greater or less epidemics during the succeeding centuries. The plague was not really conquered until the way in which it was transmitted was discovered during the nineteenth century (see page 287).

It was not, however, only the plague which terrified people during the Middle Ages. Crusaders returning from the Middle East caused the dangerous spread of leprosy. This had been a comparatively rare disease in ancient times, introduced, it is thought, by the Roman legions returning from Egypt to places north of the Alps. The incidence of leprosy was further extended as a result of the contact between Africa and Europe which the Moors maintained in Spain (see page 107). Clearly the influence of Bible stories caused a greater fear of leprosy than its epidemical importance warranted. At any rate, during the concluding years of the Crusades, towards the end of the thirteenth century when leprosy reached a dangerous rate of contagion in Europe, a feeling of panic came over the people. The result was that brutal and often inhuman measures were undertaken to fight it.

Thus the French king, Philip the Fair, who reigned from 1285 to 1314 and was famous not only for his brutal blackmail of the Jews but also for his cruel proceedings against the Order of Templars, hit on the idea of ridding the land of lepers by having them burnt to death – a significant example of what happens when a disease is regarded as a punishment from God. By a strange paradox, however, it was the Church which

127

opposed the murderous project and took the lepers into its protection. Lepers were nursed in the Holy Lazarus monasteries, which consequently became known in Europe as lazar houses. True, the monks could not protect lepers from passing the rest of their lives in a kind of living death. Lepers were cast out of human society and had to live either with other lepers in a home known as a *leprosorium,* or move to a remote dwelling which was clearly recognizable as a leper-hut by the white cross painted on it. Lepers also had to warn off healthy people by sounding a clapper.

As mentioned earlier, these measures far exaggerated leprosy's threat to public health. By the fifteenth century, no fewer than nineteen thousand homes for lepers had been founded by the religious orders of Europe. When, for no known reason, leprosy as good as vanished from this part of the world, one-and-a-half centuries later, the lazar houses became hospitals.

But plague and leprosy were by no means the only epidemics to attack people during the Middle Ages. Smallpox, a dangerous epidemic in ancient times (see page 95), had almost disappeared in Europe when it was reintroduced by the returning crusaders. For the next six centuries Europe was tormented by terrible epidemics which wrought devastation, killing millions upon millions of people.

In addition, a new and wholly unknown epidemic appeared towards the end of the fifteenth century. It was first discovered in England and was therefore known as the English sweating sickness or *sudor anglicus.* This highly contagious disease, which has to this day not been explained, began with an attack of shivering and severe generalized symptoms of illness. Then followed an outbreak of evil-smelling sweat which disappeared a few days later. The mysterious disease caused many deaths – chiefly among strong men; old people, women and children were apparently less susceptible to the English sweating sickness. In his *Chronicle of England,* Richard Grafton vividly described an outbreak of sweating sickness which took place in 1485:

... a new kynde of sicknesse came sodainely tbrough the
whole region, ... which was so sore, so paynefull and sharp,
that the like was never hearde of, to any man's rembraunce...
before that tyme. For sodainely a deadly and bourning
sweate invaded their bodies and vexed their bloud and
with a most ardent heat infested the stomacke and the head
greeuously: by the tormenting and vexacion of which
sicknesse, men were so sore handled, and so painefully pangued,
that if they were layed in their bedde, being not able to
suffer the importunate heate, they cast away the sheetes and all
the clothes lying on the bed.

Many different rumours circulated about the causes of the
mysterious English sweating sickness. Some people considered the
unhealthy English climate was responsible; others, the extraordinarily unhygienic houses and living conditions of the British;
still others the gluttony and drunkenness which men indulged in
during their banquets. At the beginning of the sixteenth century
there was another outbreak of the sweating sickness and, in 1529,
it also appeared in Hamburg, Holland, the Scandinavian countries,
Poland and Russia. Then it vanished for ever.

The tremendous burdens which the people of Europe, already
severely tested, had to bear during the Middle Ages, frequently
surpassed the limits of human endurance. The average lifespan
was short, and what most people – such as farmers, labourers,
craftsmen, bondsmen and serfs – could expect from life during
their short time on earth, was not particularly promising. Disease
and death threatened everywhere; woe betide those who were
suspected of heresy by the Church – bestial torture and burning
were certain to be their fate. Wars and robberies, besides arson
and looting committed by the powerful, could wreak ruin and
destruction over wide tracts of land and its inhabitants from one
day to the next. Cruelty and brutality committed during the
collection of taxes and ill-treatment by his superiors made the
life of the little man a living hell. Mass-poisoning from grain

which had been tainted by ergot regularly occurred, like an epidemic, and was known as St Anton's fire. Thus, the clergy did not find it hard to persuade people that life on earth was worthless and only represented a passage to a better existence in paradise.

One aspect of the incessant and unbearable fear in which man lived during the Middle Ages, was the loss of his emotional balance and the outbreak of mass panic, mass hysteria and mass frenzy, which sometimes assumed the most extraordinary and fantastic forms. Processions of flagellants traversed Europe during the middle of the fourteenth century. The flagellants, firmly convinced that the unceasing afflictions were a punishment from God, wandered through villages and towns and, twice a day, did penance in the market squares by stripping to the waist and beating themselves bloody with scourges set with iron nails. Then the 'Brotherhood of the Cross' continued on its journey.

Another form of mass frenzy was the dancing madness which caused men and women, mostly from the lower classes, to be seized by an uncontrollable compulsion which made them dance in a circle until they were in a trance and saw fantastic heavenly visions. The dance continued without pause until the dancers fell to the ground senseless and, foaming at the mouth, began to jerk like epileptics. Then the dance would begin anew and the strange thing was that, like all other cases of mass hysteria, the dancing madness attracted the bystanders with such irresistible force that they too soon began to dance and dislocate their limbs.

A final example of mass hysteria is provided by the so-called Children's Crusades which took place in 1212 from Burgundy in France and Cologne in Germany. In Burgundy, a Capuchin friar had issued an appeal for a crusade of the innocents and, at the same time, on the lower Rhine, hordes of young children crowded round a nine-year-old boy who wanted to conquer Jerusalem and the Holy Land. Like an avalanche the procession of children grew at each place it passed; nobody could stop them. Obsessed by their faith and their visions, they regarded themselves as soldiers of Christ.

The fate of both children's crusades was terrible. After the more than twenty thousand young members of the French children's crusade had wandered through the Rhône Valley, devastating it, they reached Marseilles and were embarked into seven ships by cunning speculators, ostensibly in order to reach Palestine via Egypt. As soon as they arrived at Alexandria, however, they were driven to the slave-markets and sold.

The participants of the German children's crusade fared no better. They wandered southward across difficult Alpine passes. Thousands were left behind on the wayside to starve and die. Of the twenty thousand who had set out from Cologne, only a few thousand reached the towns of Piacenza and Genoa, whence they were rapidly dispatched to Brindisi. There they waited in vain for fulfilment of the prophecy made by the friar when he had called for the crusade: for the Mediterranean to dry up so that they could continue their journey.

By the time they had realized the impossibility of their project, it was too late. The year had advanced and the Alpine passes were completely blocked by ice and snow. Of the twenty thousand children only two returned to Cologne, completely reduced by famine. When they were asked what they had hoped to achieve, they replied that they did not know.

15

The Renaissance awoke a new vital con-
consciousness. The era of discoveries.
Girolamo Fracastro and his theory of
contagious diseases. Paracelsus, a confirmed
opponent of Galen's dogmas, brought about
a turning-point in medical science.
Experience, examination and experiment
meant more to him than a belief in ancient
authorities.

While medieval Europe was still shaking with attacks of fever, while plague upon plague and epidemic after epidemic almost drove the people to despair, the spirit of humanity awoke to new ways of thinking and new experiences. Slowly and reluctantly at first, then with greater uncontrollable force, an intellectual vitality began to express itself. This consciously sought to free itself from the lifeless forms into which the medieval Church had forced every intellectual activity. Nature had been regarded as ungodly; the sinfully heathen world of antiquity had been damned and replaced by a belief in the supernatural wonder-world of Christianity. Now the first stirrings of individual, liberal thought and meditation began to make themselves felt in defiance of all the prohibitions of the clergy. A new feeling towards the world began to be experienced, a sense of individuality awoke in men who were determined to act and develop their faculties independently.

The relationship of people towards each other and towards the world was fundamentally changed. The unquestioning acceptance of an imposed and inherited system of thought no longer seemed valid. Now the fullest intellectual and emotional development of the independent spirit became the ideal of the new philosophy.

Antiquity, which until then had been rejected as 'sinful and heathen', was rediscovered and reborn. This spiritual awakening in the Renaissance has been rightly regarded as one of the great turning-points in man's intellectual development. It was a time of discoveries; the discovery of printing, by means of which new ideas were rapidly disseminated; the discovery of new lands; a new form of religion and way of looking at the world; a new system of astronomy; the rediscovery of the plastic arts and poetry of the ancients, was accompanied by a new feeling of vitality and a new concept of art; finally, the discovery and rediscovery of man himself and with this, the birth of humanism.

One place where the ancient sciences were cultivated with special affection and given new form was the old University of Padua in Northern Italy. There a spirit of freedom reigned, for Padua belonged to Venice, so its scholars dared to pursue ideas which were, at that time, regarded as highly revolutionary. Posterity has preserved the names of two members of Padua's medical faculty. Both were doctors and astronomers, both were born during the 1470s: Nikolaus Koppernigk, a Pole of German extraction who, following the humanist fashion, latinized his name into Copernicus, and Girolamo Fracastro from Verona.

Without abandoning medicine, Copernicus gave humanity the results of a daring flight of thought. His work *De Revolutionibus Orbium Caelestium* (About a new order of the heavenly spheres), a new conception of the world, which overthrew the hitherto accepted order of the constellations, proclaimed the sun as occupying the central position in the cosmic system as opposed to the Ptolemeic doctrine of the earth as centre which had been accepted until then.

Girolamo Fracastro, though he wrote poetry as well, was even more faithful to his medical calling than his fellow student, Koppernigk. After he had passed his examinations, he settled down as a doctor in a country house near Verona, surrounded by telescopes, globes and books. Contagious diseases were his special interest; he was, however, especially drawn towards a new epidemic disease which reached the Old World after Columbus returned from America. The famous explorer's sailors brought the venereal disease, syphilis, back with them from the New World. On their return they had been paid off in Barcelona. Then they decided to become mercenaries and had hurried to join the colours of King Ferdinand of Naples, who was defending his hereditary kingdom against young King Charles VIII of France. Naples surrendered after a siege lasting only three weeks; the majority of the defenders, including the Spaniards, then entered the service of the French king. They carried the odious disease with them and it spread with uncanny speed among the soldiers of the French king.

When they heard of the approach of a great imperial army to relieve Naples, the demoralized and diseased soldiers of King Charles fled north. Wherever they passed, they sowed the pernicious poison and, in no time, Italy was inundated with venereal disease. Soon afterwards it spread throughout Europe, and eventually it was to be found throughout the Old World, including North Africa and the Near East. It was no respecter of rank; emperors and kings, dukes and earls, knights, nobles, popes, cardinals, bishops and canons all had to pay the same tribute as burghers, workers, scholars and poets, monks, nuns, artisans, mercenaries, farm labourers or maidservants.

This disease, which struck at the very root of human happiness, slipping its poison between man and wife, parents and children, friend and foe, and so fouling the holiest of mankind's ties, infested whole nations. It changed energy, vitality, love of work and creative activity into hollow hopelessness and despair and brought with it a secret and, therefore, much more dreadful necessity to keep apart from other people. This disease was the subject of Fracastro's keenest research. However, he did not describe it in prosaic language but composed a didactic poem in hexameters into which he wove antique-mythological material. The conquistadores had profaned local gods during their conquest of the New World. They were punished for this with a horrible epidemic which, since time immemorial, had been haunting the native populations. How had it reached them?

A shepherd had alienated the people from their hereditary gods; the latter had avenged themselves by scattering poisonous germs into the earth, water and air. The shepherd himself was the first victim of the disease; searching for a name to call it, Fracastro borrowed from Ovid. The birthplace of Niobe, the daughter of Tantalus and wife of the Theban king, Amphion, was a hill called Sipylus near Magnesia. Niobe's second son, Sipylus, was named after the hill. Fracastro changed the name a little and called the shepherd of his poem Syphilus. The disease, from which he was the first to suffer, was called Syphilis; this originally poetic name was to remain. It was also known as the French sickness because it first appeared as an epidemic in Charles VIII of France's armies. In three volumes entitled *De Syphilide Sive de Morbo Gallico* (About syphilis or the French sickness), Fracastro described the new disease in detail, giving sensible advice for its treatment. The work was extremely favourably received – the more so as in those days only too many people were personally interested.

Girolamo Fracastro next widened the scope of his research to include other contagious or infectious diseases as well, such as plague, leprosy, erysipelas, anthrax, tuberculosis, typhus and scabies. He was the first to refer to 'specific' fevers and stated clearly and unambiguously the belief that all these diseases were called forth by an infecting agent or *contagium*. He recognized, correctly, that this infecting agent could be transmitted in three ways: either directly by physical contact from person to person; or by using objects which had been contaminated by the *con-*

tagium; or, finally, by air containing the infecting agent.

The fruit of this research was the three-volume work about contagious diseases and their treatment which appeared seven years before Fracastro's death and which, of all his works, was the most strongly pioneering. If Fracastro had been able to avail himself of a microscope and had recognized his *contagium* as being a tiny living creature, he would rightly be regarded today as the founder of the theory of infectious and contagious diseases.

While Girolamo Fracastro was comfortably re-animating the ancient spirit of research in his country house near Verona, the new spirit also began to appear in Northern Europe. During the same year, 1493, that Columbus embarked on his second voyage of discovery, a boy was born in Einsiedeln, Switzerland. He was not destined to reawaken ancient scientific ideals by leisurely meditation and research. Racked by conflict and pangs of con-science, he was restlessly driven from place to place and, as a result of his life's work, he brought about a revolution in medicine north of the Alps. His name is remembered in medical circles to this day. He was called Paracelsus.

His father came from a Swabian noble family, one of the Bombasts of Hohenheim. His mother was from Swiss burgher stock. The child was christened Theophrastus, to which his father added the nickname Paracelsus. The boy's first teacher was his father, who, a doctor by profession, took his son with him on his rounds and thus made him aware of the magnificent features of the Swiss landscape, its mountains, woods and plants.

After his mother died, when Theophrastus was ten years old, his father moved to Villach in Carinthia; and a few years later Paracelsus proceeded to the University of Ferrara to study medicine and become a doctor like his father. However, he had hardly embarked upon his studies when he, who had grown up in close contact with nature, began to experience doubts. The book-learning, which was preached from the lectern in those days, seemed to him far too ossified; he found intolerable the blind

faith in authority, which, disclaiming personal observation experience and research, uncritically accepted the stale scholastic
wisdom which had been handed down from late classical
times.

A man who was followed most uncritically of all was Galen.
This was the most decisive and revolutionary element in Paracelsus' work: he was a determined and convinced opponent
of Galen's doctrines.

Not long after he had won his doctorate at Ferrara, he cast
it light-heartedly aside, declared war on the musty book-learning
of his times and set out on his travels. He wandered restlessly
from one place to the next through the countryside – sometimes
followed by a band of dubious disciples – constantly observing,
seeking, experimenting. He felt drawn back to his father's home
in Villach, next he was to be found in Freiburg, then in Strasburg,
acquiring citizenship of the latter in 1526. After achieving one or
two sensational cures he was appointed doctor to the city during
the following year and, at the same time, he was granted the right
to hold lectures at the university.

Theophrastus' moment seemed to have come. Already, however, the revolutionary tone of the advertisement he circulated,
as was customary in those days, was not promising. 'We shall
free medicine from its worst errors. Not by following the teaching of the ancients, but by our own observation of nature, by
long practice, confirmed by experience. Who does not know that
most doctors practising today commit grave errors to the hurt
of their patients...' One is reminded of the 95 Theses which
his contemporary, Martin Luther, nailed to the door of the castle
church in Wittenberg exactly ten years earlier. Paracelsus fared
rather like that other spiritual fighter. The erudite gentlemen
of the medical faculty in Basle noted Theophrastus' programme
and took it for what it was – and what it was certainly also
intended to be – a declaration of war. The new city doctor also
dared to do something else entirely new and unheard of: he
conducted his lectures in the German language.

It was not long before the firebrand had antagonized every-one: teachers, listeners, and even the town council itself. His activities in Basle lasted just ten months. In February 1528 he was forced to flee the town, laughed at, mocked and scorned. His restless wandering life began once more. He crossed Alsace, stopped for a while in Colmar, travelled to Switzerland once again, to St Gallen, then to the Valley of the Inn, publishing books in the German language, among others: *The Great Book of Surgery*. He also wrote about syphilis, pouring biting scorn on the belief in guaiacum, a remedy which was then much in favour, saying that above all it healed the moneybags of the big merchant houses importing it.

Once more Paracelsus found recognition in his second home – Carinthia – and from there he was summoned to Salzburg. How-ever, the eternal, harassing battle he had fought had exhausted him and he died there at the early age of forty-eight.

Paracelsus, born at an exciting turning-point in Western history, gave Western medicine a new aspect. He studied nature like Hippocrates, whom he venerated above all others. His practice of paying attention to the effects of the weather, character of the ground, and general living conditions in his examination and diagnoses of disease, made him the man who reawakened and founded a scientific concept of medicine. Vital knowledge gained from life, creative experience, examination, unbiased verification and experiment were worth more to him than all the dusty, traditional authorities. It was thanks to his passion for experiment that he enlisted chemistry into the service of medicine, and he was responsible for the well-known saying: 'All things are poison, and nothing except poison; it is only the dosage which stops it being poisonous.'

The reason why Paracelsus' personality has been the subject of so much controversy may have its origin in the circumstances of his restless wandering life, with its occasional savour of char-latanism, as well as the often rather dubious character of his followers. Nevertheless, the work of this fearless and audacious revolutionary set the pace for medical science. It has special significance for medicine today and will endure for all time. The same words can be applied to this ever-restless, fanatical warrior and dynamically Faustian searcher after truth, as were spoken by his great contemporary, Luther, in 1521: 'Here I stand. I can do naught else. God help me. Amen.'

16

The human body as the 'most perfect work in creation'. Andreas Vesalius, the father of anatomical science, lays the foundation stone of the whole mighty edifice of present-day anthropology with his work: 'De Humani Corporis Fabrica'. *Anatomical studies will no longer be omitted from medical science*

The new study of scientific medicine demanded, no less than did Renaissance art, the urgent revival of anatomical knowledge. Andreas Vesalius was born into this era, on New Year's Day 1515. He was destined to reform the whole concept of anatomy, to found a new anatomical science and, by this means, also to point the way towards more efficient methods of healing. The rebirth of interest in classical art had already drawn the human body into the foreground of public attention; now, apart from one or two exceptions, it was no longer thought sinful to study it.

In his plastic art, Michaelangelo modelled the human body with accuracy and vitality which had not been known since the days of classical antiquity. Leonardo da Vinci, painter, architect, aesthete, anatomist, astronomer, physician, mechanic, builder of fortifications and many-sided inventor, was a man already advanced in years. In order to pursue his anatomical studies, he actually stole the human corpses from which he made his superb drawings. He never published these, however, but kept them secret and they were not discovered until the beginning of the present century.

Raphael, the creator of sublime paintings, was directing the construction of St Peter's in Rome when Vesalius was born. Titian, the greatest master of the Venetian school of painters, won the favour of Charles V to such an extent that he was granted the exclusive right to paint the emperor's portrait. Albrecht Dürer became the exponent of an entirely new way of looking at nature; the two Holbeins made Augsburg the centre of a new art movement in Germany.

None of these artists, who regarded the human body as being 'the most perfect work in creation', reproducing it in every position, drawing it, painting it, giving it plastic form and hewing it out of marble, were content just to know about the exterior. They did not merely wish to recreate the play of muscles and how they raised the skin. They wanted to study each and every one of those muscles and learn all about the interior of the human body.

Hesitant attempts had been made to penetrate the secrets of the construction of the human body. As a result it had been discovered that Galen, who had merely dissected pigs, monkeys, cats and dogs, had arrived at some grossly fallacious views. However, the Church had, as mentioned earlier (see page 99), endorsed the opinions of the sage of Pergamum to such a degree that it was still dangerous to point out any kind of false reasoning or mistake in his work; now, as before, the Inquisition kept a watchful eye on this.

Andreas, son of van Wesele, apothecary to the imperial court in Brussels, was animated by an uncontrollable urge to explore nature when he was only a boy. His chief interest was in the human body and the function of its organs. However, as the pursuit of such things could only be a dream for the time being, Andreas turned his thirst for knowledge towards any animal he could get hold of. He felt impelled to explore the internal anatomical construction of the creatures he examined. Soon no animal was safe from his craving for knowledge; frogs and mice, rats and squirrels, weasels and moles, even cats and dogs, had to give up their lives in order to reveal to him the internal construction of their bodies. Very neatly and properly everything was dissected and laid out. Soon the young boy's eyes were opened to the anatomical differences between the creatures he examined.

Without any hesitation, however, young Andreas went a step further. In those days, when the medieval way of thinking was still applied to so many things, execution, torture and quartering were not regarded with as much horror as they would be today. Without any fear, Andreas watched – as was possible in those days – the executions which took place on the gibbet-hill nearby and collected the bones of the victims after they had been pecked clean by ravens and bleached by the sun. It was very soon decided that he should study medicine like his grandfather, Everhardt. At the school in Louvain, the gifted young man easily learnt Latin, Greek, Hebrew, Arabic and mathematics and, when he was eighteen, he began to attend the University of Paris.

However, he was soon to be disillusioned in his hope that at this Mecca of science he would at last be able to study human anatomy and dissect human bodies to his heart's content. The learned professors did not dream of taking a scalpel into their own hands. That was considered a very menial, contemptible activity, which was left to the barbers. While the latter performed this task, the university teacher would read the corresponding section from Galen's works.

Andreas van Wesele – who, as was customary in those days, had Latinized his surname to Vesalius – very soon found out that he could learn nothing from his teachers; and then began a sinister interlude in his life. During the darkness of the night, he made his way to the cemeteries and execution grounds, unearthed the bodies which had recently been buried and secretly dissected them. He studied and studied; and the more deeply he penetrated into the secrets of the human body, the more clearly Galen's errors caught his eye. Where was the heart-bone Galen had described? Where the passage joining stomach and spleen? Where were the alleged seven individual parts of the breast-bone, where the two dividing

142

bones of the lower jaw, where the five lobes of the liver, where the connecting link between the bronchial tubes and the heart? No matter what Vesalius dissected and laid out, he was continually coming across appalling errors made by the Greco-Roman scholar. The great Leonardo had already discovered that the bronchial tubes branch out, ending in five branchlets in the lungs. He had even supported the results of his examination with an experiment. He had pumped air into the lungs and observed that, however high the pressure was, no air ever reached the heart. He had also examined the heart valves and reached the thoroughly sound conclusion that it was their function to see that the blood flowed in a certain direction.

Andreas Vesalius was able to confirm all these highly significant findings; and there came a day when he knew that Galen had never once dissected a human body in his life; he had simply applied to the human body, without seeing or checking, what he had found in the animals he had examined.

When, during the long conflict between the Habsburg empire and the French Crown, Emperor Charles V and King Francis I of France crossed swords for the third time in 1536 and the imperial troops were approaching the French capital from the Netherlands, the University of Paris was closed. At this time Andreas also turned his back on the city by the Seine; by a strange quirk of fortune, his father was attached as field dispenser to the very army of Charles V which caused Andreas to leave Paris. Vesalius returned to the town where he had gone to school and here, in Louvain, the twenty-one-year-old man received, for the first time, the permission of the university to dissect corpses and hold anatomical lectures.

However his rebellion against the doctrines of Galen, who was canonized by the all-powerful Church, soon made him an object of suspicion; when he learnt that the Inquisition was beginning to take an interest in him he hastily left the town. He travelled to Venice and in this city of artists made the acquaintance of a fellow countryman, Jan Stephan van Kalkar, who had studied painting under the great Titian. The two men continued to travel together. Their destination was Padua and, at this most famous southern university, Andreas threw himself with all his youthful ardour into the study of anatomy.

Now he really did begin a systematic exploration of the human body and very soon the first fruits of his labours began to ripen. He translated into exemplary Latin one of the tenth century medical books written by the Arabic doctor Al Rhazi (see page 110) and revised the anatomical lectures given by the Parisian professor, Winter von Andernach. Another work dating from this time demonstrates the extent to which anatomy was able to help practical medicine; it was concerned with the practice of blood-letting. In a monograph on the azygous vein Vesalius at last proved the validity of his critical reasoning, for his account of this vein, which mounts the spinal column in the pleural cavity, differs significantly from the description given by Galen.

Public recognition of Vesalius' industrious as well as distinguished activities was not long in coming. On 5 December 1537, a degree as doctor of medicine at the University of Padua was conferred on him with all the pomp usual at that time and, only days later – he was not quite twenty-three years old – he was appointed professor of anatomy and surgery.

He now had everything he needed to wrest the secrets from the human body and his zeal redoubled. As a result of his unceasing creative labours he piled discovery upon discovery and, again, it was his friend and fellow countryman, Jan Stephan van Kalkar, who loyally helped him in his work. As early as the following year, 1538, the two published an anatomical atlas with six entirely original, clear diagrams which were soon immensely popular with students. Then, in addition, a distinguished firm of publishers in Venice, who were planning to bring out a new edition of Galen's works in Latin, became aware of Vesalius and he was commissioned to revise the anatomical sections.

However, Vesalius was much more interested in his own works of discovery than in unravelling the works of the sage of Pergamum. Three months or so went by in a flash and then Vesalius had completed his real life's work. With unflagging energy he dissected and anatomized, removing layer after layer from the human body, laying out each muscle, however small, isolating the nerves and blood-vessels and exploring every inch of the intestines. Everything Vesalius found, the patient Stephan van Kalkar, under the former's constantly alert and strict supervision, conscientiously drew, painted and recorded in woodcuts. Indifferent to all the dusty and obsolete traditions he, alone, depicted what he had seen with his own eyes.

So, after hard and painfully conscientious cooperative labour, a seven-volume work on anatomy was created to which Vesalius gave the title *De Humani Corporis Fabrica* (About the workshop of the human body). Carefully supervising the production himself, he had it published in Basle in 1543. Moreover, this first systematic anatomy of the human being to be based on research and experience – which Vesalius dedicated to his ruler Emperor Charles V – was no less a landmark in the history of civilization than was the new astronomical system which Copernicus published in the same year. Vesalius' work, in which he boldly discarded every barren, obstructive and misleading authority and in which he only relied on himself and his own research, introduced a new epoch, not just for anatomical and physiological research, but for medical science in general. It ensured that anatomy would never again vanish from medicine.

However, it is only fair to remember that there were other Renaissance anatomists apart from Vesalius, who also published findings, some of which had far-reaching significance. The human organs which they were the first to describe, still bear the names of their discoverers in today's anatomical scientific nomenclature. Thus Gabriel Fallopius, who worked as an anatomist in Pisa and Padua, discovered the oviduct or fallopian tube, also the duct containing the facial nerves which runs through the temporal bone and the semicircular canals of the internal ear. Bartolomaeus Eustachius discovered the adrenal glands, the thoracic duct and the eustachian tube. Fabricius of Aquapendente was the first to see the venous valves. This discovery in particular – Fabricius was one of William Harvey's teachers (see page 170) – was to prove very important later in determining the movement of the blood in the human body.

Vesalius was just twenty-eight years old when, with his epoch-making work *De Humani Corporis Fabrica*, he laid the foundations of the whole great structure of present-day anthropology and medical science. The recognition, however, which he had confidently expected, failed to appear. He was destined to share the fate of all those who have something to give the world; colleagues, even his best friends, abused the man who had dared to cast doubts on Galen's authority. Andreas Vesalius was not thirty when he was forced to realize, full of impotent bitterness, that it was useless to try and fight the arrogant, musty, indolent and unproductive pedantry of the professors. Tired of the constant envy and malice of his own colleagues and former friends, embittered because his work was reprinted in England and Germany without first having obtained his approval, Vesalius gave up scientific research. However, that progressive man, Charles V, defying all calumnies, appointed the famous anatomist to his court. Andreas became the emperor's personal physician and, henceforward, accompanied him on his journeys.

When the emperor took up his residence in Brussels in 1546, Vesalius married Anna van Hamme, the daughter of a councillor. Once again fortune seemed to smile on the bitterly disappointed man. True, in his position as the emperor's physician he had to swallow much that was distasteful to an upright man like himself, for Charles V was anything but a gratifying patient. He suffered badly from gout, and the painful attacks only too frequently made him moody, incalculable and irascible. In addition, the emperor, who was endowed with a gigantic appetite, was especially fond of heavily spiced dishes, smoked meat, ham and bacon, salted food and herrings – in short, the very dishes his personal physician had strictly to forbid him to eat. But Charles was a stubborn patient and took little notice of Vesalius' instructions. Then, later, when the unbearable pains appeared, storms of imperial rage descended on to his personal physician. Most of all, however, Vesalius felt vexed because Charles kept up cross-connections with all kinds of charlatans and quack-surgeons and allowed himself to be talked into accepting the most outlandish remedies. The philanthropic emperor, however, ever-suspicious, tried them all out on his foot-men first.

Vesalius became more and more indispensable to the emperor who paid no heed to the back-biting and malicious ways in which some people tried to turn him against his personal physician; Vesalius' extraordinary abilities and achievements were guarantee enough that he was not bestowing his favours on an unworthy object. Vesalius, who had become the most famous doctor of his century, built a house in Brussels for himself and his fair-haired wife. The campaigns on which he accompanied his monarch ensured that his research work was not neglected under the pressures of his flourishing practice at court. They gave him plenty of opportunity to find out the nature and causes of disease by means of post-mortems. In all these ways, Andreas Vesalius proved himself to be just as competent a doctor as he had been an anatomist and, in the almanac for the year 1550, his name can be found listed among the famous men of his time – the dukes, cardinals and also the court physician, Andreas Vesalius.

When Charles V, tired and ill, retired to a monastery, handing over the sceptre to his morose son, Philip II, who was totally controlled by his confessors, this meant the end of all research by dissection of corpses. The abrupt end of a career which had begun with such hopes had arrived.

We do not know what made Vesalius suddenly leave the court in 1564 and return to Italy. It is certain that, under Philip, the Inquisition had again got its eye on him. According to tradition, he is said to have dissected a body unlawfully and suddenly noticed that he was working on a body only seemingly dead, whose heart was still beating. Thereupon he was said to have been arrested by the Inquisition and imprisoned; only Philip II's intercession on behalf of his father's personal physician saved him from the intended punishment and changed it into a vow to go on pilgrimage to Jerusalem. On his return journey, Vesalius was shipwrecked on the Greek island called Xanthe; solitary, abandoned and unknown, the greatest anatomist of all time died there of hunger and exhaustion in 1564.

17

*Greater importance given to clinical observa-
tion and knowledge gained at the patient's
bedside. Jean Fernel's 'Universal Medicine'.
The Englishman, John Caius, prepares the
ground for raising the status of the despised
guild of barbers to that of medical surgeons.
The Frenchman, Ambroise Paré, the 'father of
surgery', completes this task and creates an
entirely modern sounding 'comprehensive
treatment'.*

During the Renaissance, just as
anatomy experienced a great reform through Vesalius and his contemporaries, so the new spirit also benefited the clinical branches
of medical science. Clinical observation and knowledge gained at
the patient's bedside came more and more into their own, and
attempts to localize illnesses along pathological-anatomical lines became more pronounced. Among the many distinguished doctors of
that time some, especially, stand out, and their activities deserve to
be outlined briefly. The French court physician, Jean Fernel,
counts as one of the most important clinicians of the Renaissance.
Like so many of his colleagues he was not only a doctor of
medicine, but also a renowned mathematician and important
astronomer. However he differs favourably from other well-known
doctors of his era because he abandoned astronomy.

Jean Fernel, who lived from 1506 to 1588, published a three-part

work under the encyclopaedic title *A Universal Medicine*. To
some extent Fernel created the separate sections of his work himself; he was the first to include physiology and pathology in a comprehensive and systematic presentation, whilst the third part of his
Universal Medicine dealt with therapy. Although frequent post-
mortems carried out on patients who had died of certain diseases
led him to believe that local pathological processes were the cause
of diseases, Fernel's pronouncements, though critically opposed to
Galen, sound like humoral-pathological reflections.

Fernel enriched medical knowledge by a number of important
individual deductions, especially in symptomatology and pathological anatomy. Like all doctors of his day, he made a special study
of syphilis which he gave the scientific name *Lues venerea;* and
he examined exactly the manner in which the infection was transmitted. He was familiar with the symptoms of influenza, which he
distinguished as a separate disease and he gave interesting descriptions, based on post-mortems, of consumption and endocarditis.
In Fernel's day, there still reigned a hopeless confusion with regard
to the venereal diseases, so much so that syphilis and gonorrhoea
were regarded as different aspects of the same disease. Jean Fernel
was the first to believe that gonorrhoea was a totally different
disease from syphilis; although, it is true, his assumption only received general recognition fully three hundred years later when
his fellow countryman, Philippe Ricard, conclusively separated
gonorrhoea from syphilis.

The year 1510, exactly four years after Jean Fernel, saw the
birth in England of a man who was to prepare the way for a new
phase in medicine by raising the status of surgery. Until then, this
had been an activity which had been generally despised by the real
doctors. His name was John Caius. He had studied in Padua, as
was usual for a doctor concerned about earning his living; after
passing the examination he had settled down to practise medicine
in Norwich and later in Shrewsbury in the country of Shropshire.
His work as a doctor was crowned with such success that his fame
reached the English court and Henry VIII appointed him his court

physician. Caius made a special study of the English sweating sickness (see page 128) without, however, penetrating its secrets. His particular merit, however, was that he did not scorn to raise the status of the barber-surgeons who were despised by most other doctors and to help improve their training. Although he was by no means a surgeon himself, he did not regard it as beneath his dignity to lecture to the Guild of Barber Surgeons. He remained in favour at court even after Henry VIII's death, and Queen Elizabeth even ordained that he be granted two corpses a year for his anatomical studies. Through his endeavours to free surgeons from the Barber's Guild and raise them to the status of doctors in the best sense of the word, Caius was the forerunner of a man who, as a result of his life's work, was successful in changing the despised Guild of Barbers into the respected profession of surgical doctors.

The man to whom we are indebted for this is Ambroise Paré of France who, the fourth child of a joiner called Mattre Paré, was born in Bourg Hersant, Brittany, in 1510, the same year as John Caius. Like his brother Jean, it was decided to train the intelligent boy to become a barber and when he was thirteen he was apprenticed to a master barber called Vialet. It did not, however, give him much satisfaction to lather the stubbly faces of the Breton farmers, so he soon packed up his belongings and walked to Paris. He used the money he had saved from his apprenticeship to study at the School of Barbers, attended lectures on anatomy and was lucky enough to be numbered among the few pupils who, as a special distinction, were assigned to the Parisian hospital, the Hôtel Dieu.

He worked and studied there for three years; then, when he was twenty-six, he accompanied Marshall Montejau to the Franco-German War. Even during this first baptism of fire he proved his extraordinary surgical aptitude for treating the wounded; but a chance accident also helped to lay the foundation stone of his fame. The rules of surgery in those days laid down that, for cases of shot wounds, the passage of the wound should be bathed in boiling elder oil – clearly a dreadful torture for the wounded men. After one particularly heated conflict, Ambroise ran out of elder oil. He was reluctantly forced to abandon the usual oil treatment and instead he covered the wounds with a salve made from egg-yolks, attar of roses and turpentine.

When he visited his patients next morning he made a totally unexpected discovery. 'I saw', he himself reported, 'that those who had been treated with the salve felt only a little pain in the wound, did not suffer from any inflammation or swelling and had passed a restful night. Those, on the other hand, who had been treated with boiling oil, were suffering from fever, were in great pain and had swellings and inflammations in the region of the wound. I therefore determined never to burn the wounded in such a dreadful manner again.'

After the end of the war, when Paré was 28, he returned to Paris to complete his training, passed his examination as a barber-surgeon, married a woman by the name of Jeanne Mazelin and bought a house not far from the Seine. During the next few years he went on further campaigns as a surgeon and, in 1545, he published his first book – in clumsy French, since he knew no Latin – *The Method of Treatment for Wounds caused by Firearms*.

During further campaigns, Paré, whose fame as a surgeon was constantly increasing, reintroduced the method used by older surgeons of tying bleeding wounds with ligatures rather than the barbaric and agonizing treatment of cauterizing them. Soon his fame as the greatest surgeon of his time was such that certain jealous colleagues even made an unsuccessful attempt to poison him. In 1554, Henry II made him a master surgeon and in 1563 Ambroise published his great work *A Universal Surgery*. During the dreadful carnage of the St Bartholomew's massacre of 1572, King Charles IX saved the life of his Huguenot head surgeon by hiding him in one of the wardrobes in his dressing room. Although nothing would move the dauntless Paré, who had seen so many other people die, to renounce his faith, he nevertheless managed to remain in the king's service.

When Ambroise's wife died in 1573, he married again at the age of sixty-three and his second wife, Jacqueline Rousselet, was also a loyal companion to him. Ambroise Paré was not spared the common fate of all who made outstanding new contributions to science. The jealous members of the medical faculty, including some of his colleagues who were represented in the College of Surgeons, instituted legal proceedings against him because his books had been published without the approval of the faculty. But the king, who had appointed Paré to the royal council, was able to quash the wretched proceedings.

A rich and fulfilled life came to an end when Paré died in his eightieth year on 20 December 1590. His name cannot conceivably be left out of any history of medicine. The artisan's son who did not even know Latin – unthinkable for a scientist of those days – the former barber, through his work gave the first impetus to advance the position of the Guild of Barbers to that of medical surgeons. By his skill, personality and the maxim he consistently followed: 'surgery is learnt with the eyes and the hands', he achieved the foundation of the Royal Surgical College. Just as Andreas Vesalius was justly called 'the father of anatomy', so Ambroise Paré deserves to be known as 'the father of surgery'.

Nevertheless, it would be less than justice if this great medical pioneer were only to be remembered as the founder of scientific medical surgery. In the care and healing of his patients Paré put into practice highly modern ideas and a comprehensive form of treatment which has only come into its own in our day. He was convinced that a patient who was at odds with himself and who did not believe in the possibility of a cure, would never get well. Also that it was, moreover, of decisive significance to strengthen the patient's will to be cured in every possible way, and instill into him courage and confidence in his medical practitioner; this quite apart from treating him with a specific therapy. Hence, he was not just concerned to heal wounds and fractures but, during his treatment, bothered about every trifle, saw to it that his patients did not become bored and therefore nervous, but was anxious to alleviate the tedium of their convalescence by all kinds of suitable recreation.

At one time, when the king had commanded him to treat the Marquis d'Aurel, who some months earlier had suffered a double fracture of the thigh which would not heal, he recognized at once that splinters of bone had been left in the wound; he provided a means of escape for the pus and immediately the condition of the marquis improved.

He did not, however, regard his medical duties as over yet. He wrote: 'When I saw that my patient was slowly beginning to feel better, I told him to listen to the music of violins and violas and to send for a buffoon to make him laugh. He really did laugh and only a month later he was able to sit up in a chair and let himself be carried into his garden . . .' After this, Ambroise Paré, who had also made himself familiar with the construction of artificial flexible limbs, was successful in effecting a total cure.

The Frenchman, Guillaume de Baillou, was born a good quarter of a century after John Caius and Ambroise Paré. He added a number of valuable individual discoveries to the clinical medicine of the Renaissance and his work reflects the progress which medical science made during his times. He, too, worked on the treatment of the still highly topical disease, syphilis, and pondered the riddle of the English sweating sickness which had still not been solved (see page 128).

A great many different kinds of infections were given the generic name 'fever' in those days; Guillaume de Baillou differentiated for the first time between malaria, typhus, scarlet fever and chicken-pox. He was the first to describe the symptoms of whooping cough. He follows Hippocrates in his observations on the cause of epidemics. He is even familiar with mountain sickness.

The clinical advances of that time were due, in no small measure, to a discovery of one of the most important teaching aids in practical medicine; the teaching of medical students round the sick-bed. This practice was especially widely used in the North Italian centre of Renaissance medicine, Padua. From there it also spread north to the University of Leiden in the Netherlands.

An account of Renaissance medicine would be incomplete without mentioning one of the most important subjects subsidiary to healing: Botany. One of its chief exponents was the naturalist, Konrad Gesner, who was born in Zürich in 1516 and who was justly called the German Pliny. He was, like so many great minds of his time, an all-round genius: doctor, physician, literary historian, zoologist, botanist, and mineralogist. He raised botany to the level of a science.

In Germany, it was Valerius Cordus, born in Erfurt in 1515, who pioneered the science of botany, identified five hundred new species of plants and, with his *Dispensatorium Pharmacorum Omnium, quae in usu Potissimum Sunt* (Pharmaceutical book of all useful medicinal plants), created the first pharmacology to be used in Germany. These advances were extremely important as herbal remedies were widely used at that time.

Had not Ambroise Paré taught that surgery must not be learnt from books but by means of hands and eyes? Had not Paracelsus proclaimed that the traditional 'classics' were a positive brake on progress in medical science and that the doctors of his day would do better to study in the big book of nature? Now the words of Roger Bacon, written more than three hundred years earlier, came into their own: 'Experimental science has three great advantages over all other sciences; it discovers truths which would never otherwise be found; it examines the course of nature and it makes possible knowledge of the past and of the future.'

Thus, all the conditions necessary for the medical progress and revolutionary discoveries of the coming centuries were accomplished.

Before discussing these, however, mention must be made of a dreadful aberration of the human spirit which was particularly widespread during the Renaissance. This was witch-hunting. If people living today had not experienced something very similar, they might have found it hard to understand how the birth of such a grim superstition could happen at a time when the human spirit was soaring to such unique, immortal heights.

18

*Heresy and the Inquisition. The Church's fight
against devils, magic and witches. The inhuman
witch-trials and the true mainsprings of the
persecution of heretics and witches. Johannes
Weyer and his courageous battle against the
spiritual epidemic of witch-mania.*

The Renaissance was a period full of contradictions and paradoxes. While the ancient skills and sciences were putting out glorious new blossoms, violence and murder, cruelty and inhumanity, dagger and poison were rife. Heavenly beauty was confronted by horror, the intellect by bestiality. The era of humanism was anything but humane; the beginnings of public hygiene, created during the plague epidemics (see page 126) had already been forgotten again. Never had the city streets been so indescribably filthy as during the Renaissance; never did superstition and bloodthirstiness put out such abundant, poisonous flowers as during that time of overwhelming artistic creation and intellectual achievement. Whoever may think that the days of mass hysteria and frenzy, described in Chapter 14, had come to an end when this era of intellectual revival began, will change his mind when he considers the witch-mania that began during the Renaissance and continued for a good three hundred years.

It began with the foundation of the Cathar sect (or purists) on the Balkan peninsula and the Waldensian sect, established by the merchant, Petrus Waldus of Lyons. The Cathars wanted to re-surrect the pure, fundamental teaching of Christ, the Waldensians were also dissatisfied with the existing Catholic Church and de-manded the restoration of the original purity of Christian belief. Both sects soon spread across Italy, France and Bohemia and – as was only to be expected – the Church was afraid of the large fol-lowing which the 'heresies' were attracting. The word 'Cathar' become *gazzan* in Italian and the German word for heretic, *ketzer*, was derived from this (though the English word 'heretic' comes from the Greek *hairetikos* or one who chooses). During the years to come, the term 'heresy' came to be applied to everything that displeased the Church. The sectarians were attacked with almost unparalleled brutality; the towns and villages in which they lived were razed to the ground; men, women and children pitilessly slaughtered.

In the Dominican Order, the Pope found a congregation which devoted itself, with exemplary zeal, to the extermination of heresy. The Inquisition was established and torture introduced. The Dominicans were delegated to carry out these procedures and, as a result, they acquired almost supreme power. They did not con-cern themselves with worldly justice; all measures were justifiable in cases where heresy was suspected.

Because of their constant pursuit of heresy, the Dominicans who, like the secret police centuries later, were accountable to no one, formed a regular state within the state. It was they who, by means of their passionate sermons in village and town, by their broadsheets and proclamations, systematically bred such a belief in devils, demons, the black arts and witches in people's imagina-tions, that they thought they saw the hand of the devil in every un-usual incident.

An unprecedented psychosis took hold of the people; even those belonging to the intellectual, civilized ranks of society were over-come by the manic belief in devils and demons which was to continue to hold sway over men's minds for centuries to come. It is scarcely credible but true that, whereas in AD 500, a belief in demons and devils was regarded as a wicked regression into heathendom, almost a thousand years later the everlasting circle of events caused a profoundly new belief in magic, demons and witchcraft to grow up which was to equal that of the worst era before classical antiquity.

The Church declared bitter war on devils, magic and witches; in 1448 Pope Innocent VIII issued his bull *Summis Desiderantes Affectibus*, summoning the clergy to exercise no mercy in their pursuit of heresy but to use the harshest measures to destroy it. Sectarianism, heterodoxy, magic and witchcraft soon became merged into a single concept and out of this amalgam of mania and superstition, a figure was formed which was presented to the people as public enemy number one: the witch.

Generations of people have tried to discover why the female sex should have been accused of being the personification of all evil beside, or in connection with, the devil. Passages can be found in the Bible which can be interpreted in this sense. For example, there is a passage in *Ecclesiasticus* which suggests that the evil of the world is but slight compared with that of woman and that as sin came first from a woman it is because of woman that we all must die.

In the same book, *Ecclesiasticus*, however, there are also many eulogies on virtuous, good and tender women. It therefore seems positively absurd to make use of the Bible as a *carte blanche* for the persecution of witches. The real reason why witch-mania was artificially stimulated, why even the writings of Thomas Aquinas were drawn on in an attempt to justify such persecutions, lie on an entirely different plane. The Church had to set to work with all zeal to restore its absolute sovereignty, for ominous cracks had begun to appear in its fabric. What does a state do when it sees danger approaching? It throws down the tastiest possible morsel before the masses.

This long-established recipe was followed then. The Order of Dominicans took to its macabre task more quickly than expected; the Church's *coup d'état* – as a theologian described the Inquisition – had succeeded. Perhaps the unbiased reader may ask what connection there is between witch-hunting and the evolution of medical science. However, the whole phenomenon which Gustav Schenk described as 'the greatest epidemic in Western, and probably even world, history' is such a unique example of mass psychosis and delivered so many millions of people to the most agonizing of all deaths, that it deserves just as much attention as the epidemics of earlier centuries.

The persecution of witches was reduced to a simple and straightforward system when the inquisitors, Heinrich Krämer and Jacob Sprenger wrote *The Hammer of Witches* (*Malleus Maleficarum*), which appeared in 1487. It has been justly called 'the most pernicious testimony in all the world's literature'. In the 650 printed pages was set out, in three sections, which kind of people should count as witches, what kinds of bewitchment there were, and how the extermination or punishment should be effected by the temporal or spiritual court. A translator called the book 'an incredible monster filled with an intellectual stench' and decided that 'in the arguments which in his view bordered on stupidity, but a stupidity shot with theological pride, a cold-blooded, idle cynicism supervened, a wretched and contemptible predilection for tormenting people which constantly reawakens the reader's wrath and uttermost bitterness over this monstrous religious mania.'

The more the witch-trials gained ground, the more plainly was revealed the motivating force which should already have been apparent, reading between the lines, in *The Hammer of Witches*. This was the unbridled, habitual sadism, a perverted bloodlust, of the inquisitors, and a bestial delight in tormenting people – especially when the victims were of the female sex. This was what happened: before the offenders were brought in for torture, they were bathed; in some places their hair was also dressed, and then, as prescribed in *The Hammer of Witches*, they were stripped in order to discover whether any kind of witch's instrument had been sewn into their clothes – instruments which they were frequently supposed to have been taught by demons to make from the bones of an unbaptized boy. As a further precaution, *The Hammer of Witches* also prescribed that the hair should be shaved from every part of the body for the same reason as the removal of the clothes had been recommended. 'For they have sometimes, in order to further their witchcraft, hidden some superstitious amulet made of certain things, either among their clothes or the hair of their body and sometimes even in the most secret, unmentionable places.'

After she had been prepared in this way, the 'witch' was laid naked on a bench for examination and every part of her body, however concealed, subjected to the most embarrassingly exact scrutiny, in the search for a witch-sign. Such things as moles, warts and the like were counted as witch-signs; red hair was itself highly suspicious. That the whole procedure only served to satisfy the perverse titillation of the inquisitors is best shown by the fact that the outcome was always the same, no matter what the examination revealed. If the *stigma diabolicum* was found it was a sure sign of the victim's relationship with the devil; if it was missing, this was an even more conclusive proof for the devil could naturally be expected to protect his strumpet.

The enormities to which the inquisitors ventured can be seen by the fact that young girls were even examined to see if they were virgins. Here again, however, the results made no difference to the sequel. If the girl proved to be a virgin it was argued that the devil had induced this condition in order to please his strumpet. If the young girl was no longer a virgin, she must naturally have had intercourse with the devil.

Hardly anyone was safe from the clutches of the Dominicans. In Würzburg, for example, the following types of people were tried for witchcraft and, after torture, executed: the daughter of a noble chancellor, a goldsmith's wife, a midwife, the wife of a provost of the cathedral, the wife of a councillor, a twelve-year-old foreign girl, a councillor, a middle-class woman and her daughter, a rich man, a mother with both her infant daughters, a young twenty-four-year-old girl, a schoolboy, two noble boys, the two daughters and maid of a town bailiff, the chemist's wife and her daughter, a fifteen-year-old girl, another young girl, the most beautiful young girl in Würzburg, etc., etc.

In the innumerable records of trials preserved from those dark times, the facts are always the same: the accused had to state that they had had intercourse with the devil. They had to describe in every detail exactly what they had experienced and, in order to get these statements from them, they were subjected to the most horrible tortures which a perverted mind could imagine.

Many confessed; but it is hard to decide today whether they really believed what they said or whether they merely preferred to die than go on being scourged, whipped, subjected to the thumb-screws or Spanish boot, have their limbs dislocated, crushed or torn on the rack, their bodies filled with water or be drawn up by their hands – which had first been tied behind their backs – and then dropped, suddenly – or whatever other satanic methods of torture were devised.

Moreover, the inhuman torments which the victims were re-peatedly made to endure, helped provide the inquisitors with fresh material. When the agony was at its height, the inquisitors would dangle before their victims the prospect of mercy if they would name accessories, accomplices or other 'witches'. In order to escape further torture, the desperate creatures must often have murmured the name of some acquaintance or even relative. However, it was more than enough for a new prosecution; denunciation, mere suspicion even, was enough on which to base an action which brought a whole string of others in its train.

There were, it is true, beside the sadistic perversions of the in-quisitors, other motives for the inhuman processes against witches and warlocks. Many a personal act of enmity, many a deed of revenge, may have been performed in this terrible way; and finally, there existed a third motivating force: money. The greatest care was taken to note the taxable value of their property in the documents on the person under suspicion. If anyone, man or woman, was wealthy, he was already doomed for if, as the result of a denunciation, he was put to the question and a 'confession'

1. Babylonian seal engraved with healing deities and medical instruments. *Louvre*, Paris

2. Bronze figure of Imhotep. *British Museum*, London

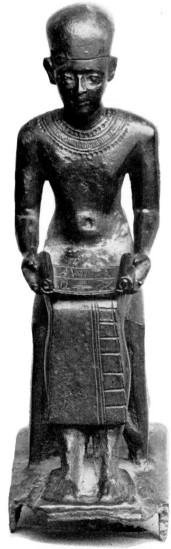

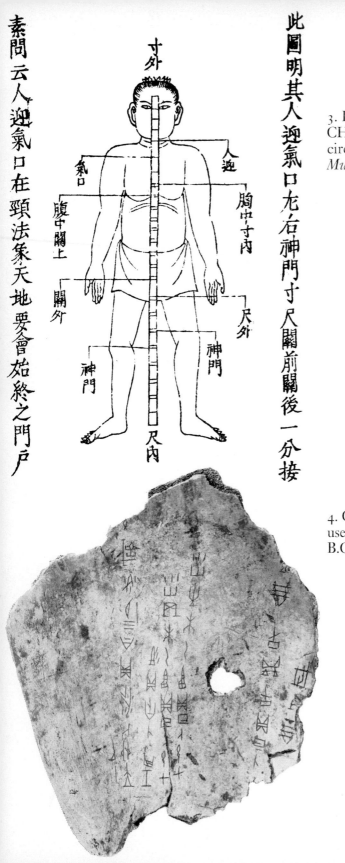

素問 云人迎氣口在頸法象天地要會始終之門戶

此圖明其人迎氣口左右神門寸尺關前關後一分接

寸外
人迎
氣口
胸中寸內
腹中關上
尺外
關外
神門
神門
尺內

3. Illustration from NAN-CHING (Theory of Pulse), circa A.D. 1500. *British Museum*, London

4. Carved bone from China, used as oracle, circa 1600 B.C. *British Museum*, London

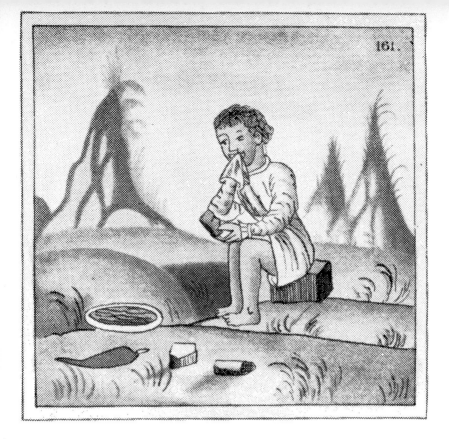

5. 'Cleaning Teeth' and 6. 'Treatment of Fever'. Illustrations from sixteenth century Florentine Codex by Fra Bernardino de Sahagun, translated from Aztec into English. *University of Utah*, U.S.A.

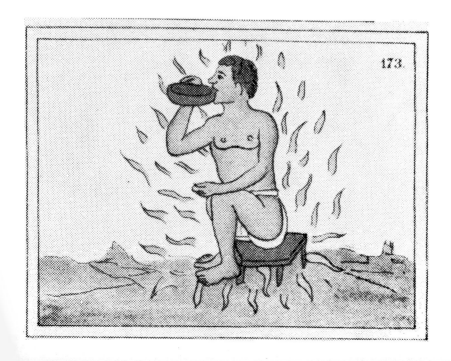

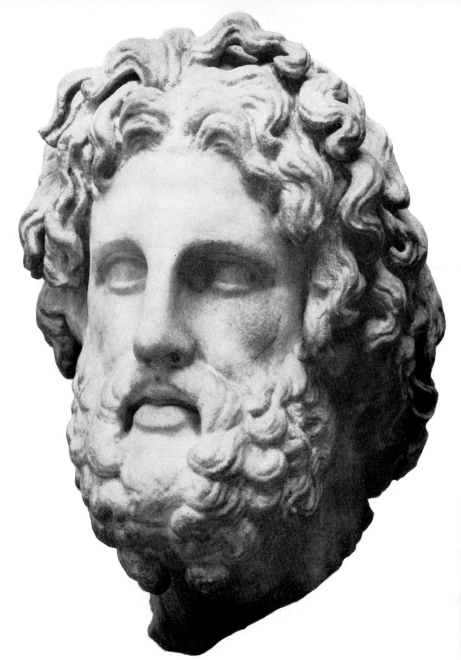

7. Statue of Aesculapius (from Melos, about 300 B.C.). *British Museum*, London

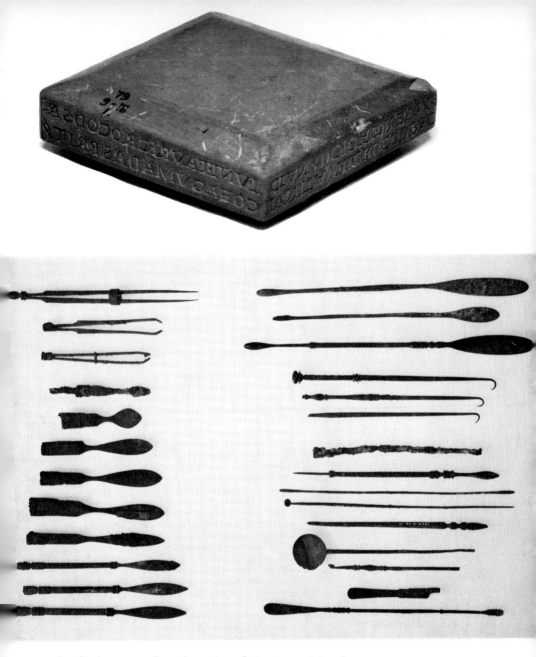

8. Oculist's stamp, thought to be of Roman origin, first century A.D. *British Museum*, London

9. Surgical instruments. Roman, first century A.D. *British Museum*, London

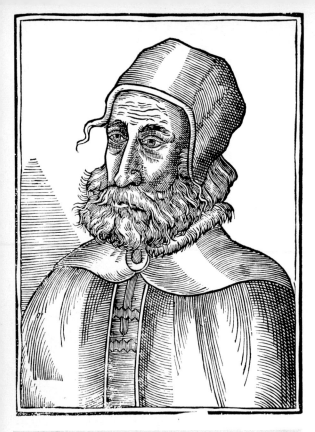

10. Galen (Claudius Galenus),
c. A.D. 130–200. Woodcut
reproduction from a copy
of Bon. Gra. Paris Med.,
in the possession of the
Royal College of Physicians,
London

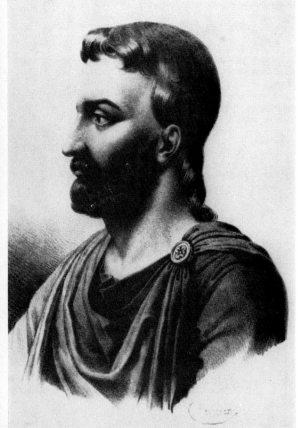

11. Celsus (Aurelius
Cornelius), 25 B.C. – A.D.
50. Engraving by Vigneron.
Royal College of Physicians,
London

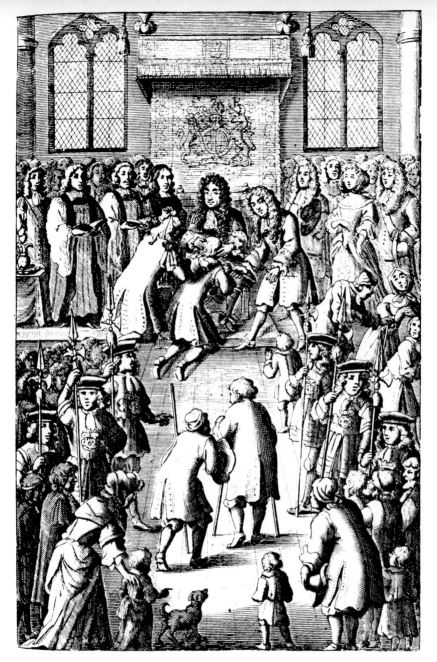

12. Curing the King's Evil. Illustration from John
Browne's ADENOCHOIRADELOGIA, 1684. *British
Museum*, London

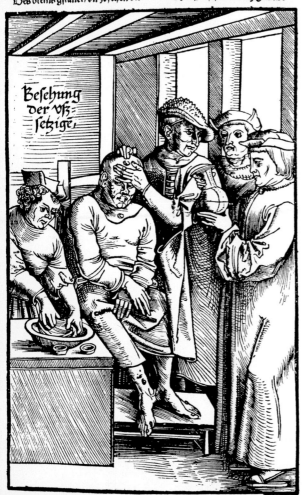

Blůt/harn/knoll/drůßen/glyder fůl/
Des otems gstanck/vñ zeychen vil

Für wot red ich/die zßigen an/
Dz dißer sey ein malzigman.

Beschung
der vß=
setzige.

13. Medieval treatment of
scabies. From an engraving
in the possession of the
Staatsbibliothek Berlin,
(*Archiv Handke*)

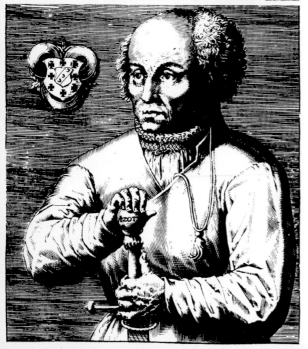

14. Paracelsus (Aurelius
Philippus Theophrastus),
1493–1541. From a copy of
BIBLIOTHECA
CHALCOGRAPHICA by
Boissart in the possession
of the *Royal College of
Physicians*, London

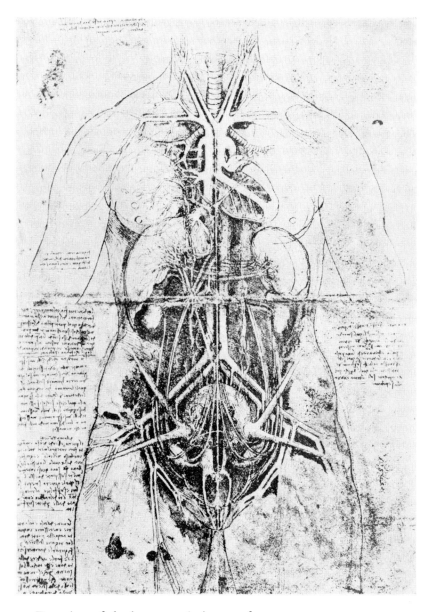

15. Drawing of the breast and viscera of a pregnant woman by Leonardo da Vinci. *Staatsbibliothek Berlin (Archiv Handke)*

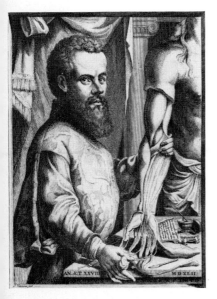

16. Portrait of Vesalius by Calcar, reproduced in DÉ RADICIS CHINAE USU EPISTOLA by Vesalius, published 1546. From a copy in the possession of the *Royal College of Physicians*, London

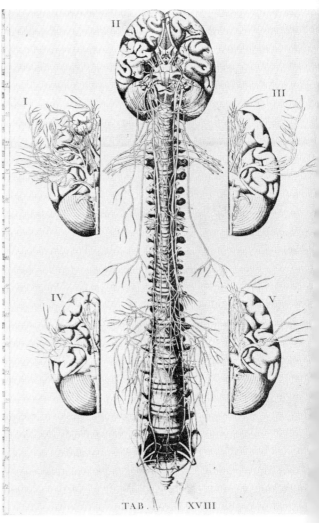

17. Drawing of the nervous system according to Bartolomeo Eustachius. *Staatsbibliothek Berlin (Archiv Handke)*

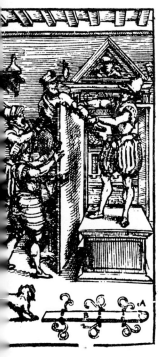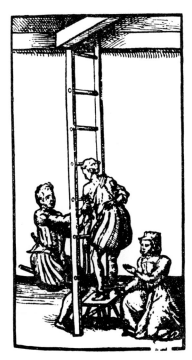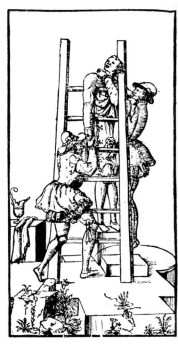

19. Engravings: 'Methods of straightening limbs' from
OEUVRES DE M. AMBROISE PARE published in 1573
by Gabriel Buon

18. Engraving of an artificial
hand from OEUVRES
DE M. AMBROISE PARE
published in 1573 by
Gabriel Buon

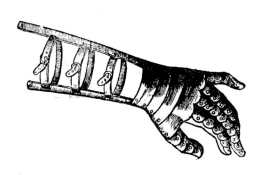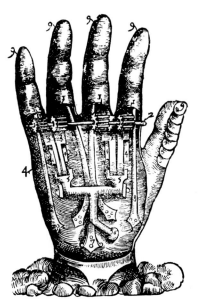

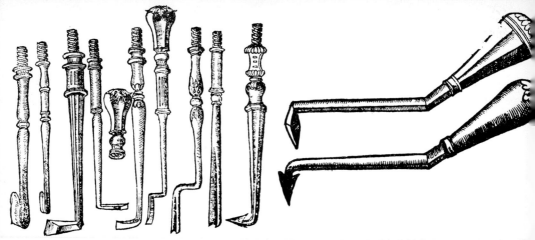

20. Surgical instruments illustrated in OEUVRES DE M. AMBROISE PARE published in 1573 by Gabriel Buon

21. Animal/human blood transfusion following Harvey's discovery of the circulation of the blood. Illustration from a book by M. G. Purmann in the possession of the *Staatsbibliothek Berlin* (*Archiv Handke*)

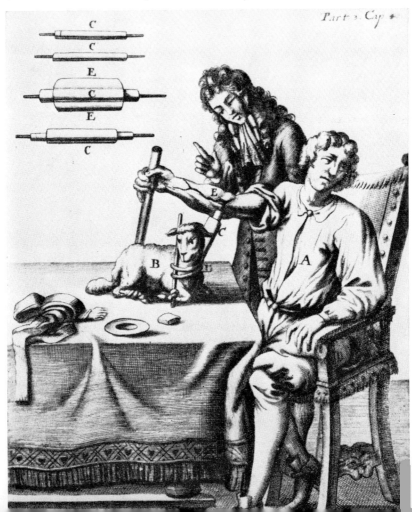

extracted from him under torture, his property was liable to be confiscated as soon as sentence had been passed on him by the court. Two-thirds of his property would go to the public treasury, the remaining third would be divided among judge, inquisitors, denunciators, torturers and executioner.

The number of victims claimed by the witch-hunts, which lasted for three hundred years, is reckoned by historians to be between five and six million people; it therefore caused more deaths than all the wars waged over that period. People today may find it hard to understand how civilized people could put up with having their nearest relatives imprisoned, tortured, and finally burnt alive, as a result of an anonymous denunciation.

It is only when one takes into account the brutal, pitiless, expression of mass mania, and that a belief in the devil, his traffic with witches and warlocks, was constantly being fanned anew by the Church and exhortations to fight them passionately proclaimed, that it is possible to gain any measure of understanding of the horror-inspiring mixture of religion and brutality, fervour and fear, lasciviousness and outrage which reigned over people in those times.

Many questions, however, remain unanswered; and it seems baffling that the sexual urge should have become transformed into bloodthirsty sadism in such a great number of people. After all, there is hardly one sphere of human life that is so full of mysteries as the sexual urge. The fact that it is impossible to imagine Ancient Greece without homosexuality strikes the person of today as scarcely less strange than the bloodlust and routine sadism of the inquisitors.

What the 'witches' – according to the trial reports – said about their relationship with the devil is, however, just as full of mystery. Leaving aside the 'confessions' extracted under torture, a great number of self-accusations remain to give one pause for thought. W. Lindenberg connects the devil experiences which many witches freely volunteered with the magic potions which were in common use at that time. In every farm garden grew such *solanaceae* as henbane, belladonna, mandrake (*Mandragora officinalis*), Japanese belladonna (*Scopolia japonica*) and stramonium; the 'alkaloid' contents of which, being either euphoric or intoxicating in effect, were used by medieval man as a stimulant. Hemlock and aconite completed the list of plants which induced conditions of ecstasy. Extract of henbane was even added to the ale which men drank every day.

It is not hard to see that people, especially women, who were living in an atmosphere of hellfire, demons and devilry which was constantly being stirred up again by sermons, broadsheets and pamphlets, should, under the influence of hallucinatory drugs, imagine they were genuinely experiencing something devilish and testify accordingly. Frustrated females availed themselves of the services of 'wise women' dealing in love-potions and magic salves in order to achieve the required result, and many of them probably made the voluntary confessions which the witch-trials mention.

The first people who courageously took up the fight against the mass hysteria of witch-hunting, were the famous humanists Cornelius Agrippa of Nettesheim and Johannes Weyer, a doctor from Cleves, who was born in 1515 in the town of Grave on the River Maas south of Nijmegen. At the age of seventeen, Johannes Weyer became a student of Agrippa in Bonn. The latter was an enlightened man, far in advance of his times, who often poured scorn on the pig-headedness and superstition of the clergy. It was from him that Johannes Weyer learnt to detest the madness of the witch-trials, the barbarous tortures, the ordeals by fire and water and, last but not least, the stake.

After Johannes Weyer had spent two years in Bonn making his master Agrippa's ideas his own, he studied medicine in Paris and Orleans and, when he was twenty-two, he graduated there as a doctor of medicine. He proved himself a competent clinician during his work in the Paris hospitals, and produced excellent descriptions of the English sweating sickness, scurvy, and that congenital malformation of the female reproductive organ which is called haematocolpos and which causes the menstrual blood to collect in the vagina when there is no passage through which it can escape.

Weyer's greatest service, however, consisted of his opposition to the witch-hunt with all the eloquence at his command, and, undeterred, he courageously expressed the opinion that witches were not the devil's strumpets but unfortunate mental cases. He also pointed out that the words in *Exodus* 'Thou shalt not suffer a witch to live' (*Exodus* 22 : 18) – which had provided the original pretext justifying the witch-trials – were based on a false translation for the Hebrew word *Kasaph* did not mean witch but poisoner.

Promoted to the position of personal physician to the tolerant and intelligent William III, Duke of Juliers-Cleves-Berg, Johann Weyer spent his spare time writing a book about folly and superstition. The words he wrote in the foreword, about the disgrace of witch-hunting, were at that time extremely brave. 'Almost all theologians are silent in the face of this godlessness; the doctors suffer it, the lawyers practise it, caught fast in prejudice. Wherever I go there is no one, no one who out of pity for humanity reveals the labyrinth, or raises his hand to heal the deadly wound. So I have taken over this heavy matter which disgraces our Christian faith with my humble service to dare . . .'

But centuries were to pass before Johann Weyer's brave act found its full reward. After the madness of the witch-hunts had reached its height during the seventeenth century, men appeared who, by word and deed, set themselves against the most destructive and most abominable spiritual epidemic of mankind. Friedrich von Spee-Langenfeld, Jesuit priest, divine, poet and professor in Cologne, Paderborn, Würzburg, Peine and Trier, became a benefactor of mankind as a result of his brave battle against the burning of witches in the first quarter of the seventeenth century; but again more than a century was to pass before documents relating to witch-trials gradually disappeared from criminal proceedings.

It was not until the middle of the eighteenth century, that common sense began to triumph over the madness and the spiritual epidemic, which had afflicted people for three hundred years, began to die away. Opposition to the delusion grew stronger everywhere; people began to feel ashamed of the witch-hunts and the crime of witchcraft was removed from the statute book. The last official trials for witchcraft were held in 1754 and 1756 in Landshut, Bavaria, and in 1782 a servant girl was executed for witchcraft in Glarus, Switzerland. In 1836, however, on the Hela peninsula, a young woman was put to the witch-test, found guilty and drowned.

19

*The Spanish doctor, Miguel Serveto, the
unlucky victim of Calvin, the religious despot
of Geneva, discovers the lesser or pulmonary
circulation. The Englishman, William Harvey,
solves the mystery of the greater or systematic
circulation. A new system of physiology,
based on scales and measurements, joins
descriptive anatomy.*

It would be wrong to assume
that the witch-mania was restricted to the Roman Catholic world.
The Reformation took over the abominable superstitious belief
in demons and witches lock, stock and barrel, with torture and
with stake. Also – hard though it is to understand but nevertheless
true – a man with both feet planted as firmly on the ground as
Martin Luther believed in the actual existence of Satan. In his
Tabletalk there is the following obscure sentence: 'Satan lays
changelings and people with goitre in place of the genuine child in
order to plague people. He drags sundry girls into perdition,
making them pregnant and keeping them by him until the child is
born.'

There were other Protestant reformers, however, who were to
varying degrees zealous in the destruction of heretics; John Calvin
was of their number. He managed to set up a regular secret police
with a whole army of informers, agents, searchers and myrmidons
in the city state of Geneva which he ruled with draconian severity.

During the period from 1542 to 1546 alone, he had fifty-eight people executed who offended against his ecclesiastical discipline, often for the most trifling offences; an immense number of young people were flung into prison and tortured. In the dark seclusion of his tyrannical faith, and his narrow-minded totalitarian claim, as God's dictator, to all things religious, Calvin was quite incapable of reading the signs of the times.

So, among his victims, there was also the Spanish scholar, Miguel Serveto de Reves, whose name is inscribed for all time in the golden book of medicine. Serveto, a pupil of Jean Fernel (see page 149) and a fellow-student of Andreas Vesalius and Ambroise Paré, discovered – almost a century before William Harvey – the lesser or pulmonary circulation of the blood.

Serveto, who was primarily a doctor, but also a geographer, mathematician, astronomer, and scholar of the Church, came to the conclusion, during his anatomical studies at the University of Paris, that the pores in the dividing wall of the heart, postulated by Galen, and affirmed mechanically by everyone since, did not exist. Quite clearly and unmistakably, he expressed his views about the movement of the blood between heart and lungs.

That vital spirit, the arterial blood, leaves the lungs laden with strength, heat, air, water and fire and enters the left ventricle. The vital spirit is formed as a result of the mixing of air in the lungs with the blood which reaches the lungs from the right ventricle and is afterwards hurled into the left ventricle. This connection is not made across the wall of the heart, but very cunningly: the blood is pumped out of the right ventricle and conducted to the lungs. The lungs make the blood bright and fresh, and then, via the arteries it is passed to the veins, from which it is pumped into the left ventricle and so reaches all the arteries in the body.

In view of the last words of this explanation, in which only the word 'oxygen' is missing – it was only discovered two centuries later by an Englishman called Priestley and a chemist from Stralsund called Scheele (see page 213) – it is very probable that

Serveto was also aware of the greater or systematic circulation of the blood which William Harvey was later to discover anew. Serveto was also in general a progressive doctor; he rejected the then customary indiscriminate use of purges and gave useful recipes for the preparation of medicines.

Apart from medicine and the other sciences, Serveto had an unfortunate passion for occupying himself with theological questions and this was to have disastrous effects for the young firebrand. In 1531 the young twenty-year-old man, who was as talented as he was versatile, had published a work about the errors of the trinitarian entity, as taught in the Protestant Church, in which he rejected the dogma of the so-called trinity and instead postulated three 'dispositions' of the one, indivisible and eternal God. Twenty years later, he published a further theological work: *De Christianismi Restitutione*, in which he shed critical light on the Bible.

With a mixture of blind confidence and frivolity which is hard to understand, he sent a copy of the book to Calvin so that he might discuss, with the famous champion of Protestant teaching, the questions which had deeply moved him. However, he met with inflexible resistance from the despotic religious leader in Geneva. As far as he was concerned, anyone who did not swear to every last detail of the Calvinistic dogma was a lost soul and his thoughts about Serveto, with whom he had already been in correspondence before publication of the *Restitutione*, can be seen most clearly from the words written by Calvin in which that humane man of God judged Serveto: 'This limb of Stan prevents me from more important matters .. if this creature ever dares to visit Geneva, he shall not leave that town alive.'

The foolhardy man in fact did take the risk. Since the dictator could not lay hands on Serveto, he, who was normally such a bitter opponent of the Catholic Church, by an unparalleled act of betrayal denounced Serveto to the Catholic Inquisition, attaching to his denunciation all the material he could find, including the personal correspondence. As a result, Serveto was arrested in Lyons, but since he was remarkably badly guarded, he succeeded in escaping. He hid in a Cistercian monastery but, three months later, it seemed as if an irresistible urge was driving him into danger. In July 1553 he travelled to Geneva and put up in a little-known inn. He was recognized, however, and soon Calvin, without showing a flicker of Christian pity, was able to give full rein to his wrath. Serveto was thrown into a dark, gloomy prison cell and kept there for three months, during which time he was subjected to the most unspeakable bodily and mental agonies. He begged to be allowed someone to defend him at his forthcoming trial, but that man of God, Calvin, replied mockingly: 'So great a liar needs no defence.'

Serveto's trial took place on 27 October 1553 and he was condemned to be burnt at the stake immediately afterwards. On his way to the execution ground, the broken man begged to be put to death by the sword rather than the fire, but his prayers fell on deaf ears. The merciless fanatic ordered the deeply religious Serveto to be burnt to death as slowly as possible in damp straw.

Nobody studying Miguel Serveto's works will have much doubt that Serveto at least sensed the existence of the greater circulation. It seems all the stranger, therefore, that the spark did not catch fire. The time was not yet ripe, however, and whereas Johannes Kepler had already been able to work out the exact course of the planets, the most extraordinary ideas were prevalent about the movement of the blood in a human body.

Another successor of Vesalius to the chair of anatomy in Padua, Girolamo Fabrizio d'Aquapendente, did not succeed either. He saw and described the valves of the blood-vessels but how does he describe them? 'Pocket-like' arrangements whose function it is to hold the blood which would otherwise 'collect in the extremities'.

At the turn of the seventeenth Century, one of Fabrizio's students was the Englishman, William Harvey; and this time the pupil was to surpass his master. Today it is hard to decide whether the ideas which made Harvey such a pioneer of physiological research first came to him in Padua or only later, after returning home.

To begin with, it is true, there was nothing to indicate the great deeds to come. Padua's traditional scholasticism, continuing the ancient legacy of Alexandria, held him fast for four whole years Harvey's student days ended when he received his doctor's degree and, in 1602, when he was twenty-four years old, he returned to London.

Swiftly, as a result of his abilities, he built up a big, lucrative practice; he became a hospital doctor and soon the saying, 'A doctor either has no time to eat or he has nothing to eat' could be said to apply to this busy man. But however much Harvey hurried from one sick-bed to the next, saw patients in his consulting rooms, looked after the sick in hospital, he was like a person drawn back to the sunshine and palms he has once known, drawn back to the ideas on physiology which he had imbibed in Padua. It was, in particular, the movement of the blood in the body which had captivated him since his student days in Italy.

He constantly pondered Galen's theories which still remained unaltered, according to which food which had been transformed into blood in the liver was sent to the right half of the heart by the pulsations of the blood-vessels; from here it streamed into the left chamber of the heart through the pores in the dividing wall of the heart and was then sent into the rest of the body by the spasms created by the heart muscles, by the pulse, without returning.

Just as a single flash of lightning can illuminate the whole country-side on a dark night, so a single idea started the whole well-constructed edifice of Galen's theories to totter before William Harvey's eyes, and made him conceive of an entirely new way in which the blood might move in the body. As the result of one question, Galen's theories collapsed like a house of cards: *how much* blood is sent into the body after each spasm of the heart?

Harvey could not get away from this question, and it must have been a mania for research which made him spend every free minute away from his manifold duties as a doctor investigating the movement of the blood. He pondered, calculated, dissected, vivisected; examined the heart and system of blood-vessels of no less than 128 different animals; and finally his studies permitted him to answer the question of how much blood is sent into the body with each heartbeat. After a vast number of comparisons he calculated the amount for a human being to be 60 cubic centimetres; his calculations are confirmed by modern scientific tests which show that the output of the heart is between 40 and 100 cubic centimetres.

Harvey went on calculating: the heart contracts between 60 and 80 times every minute; between 4 and 5 litres are therefore sent down into the body every minute and between 250 and 270 litres in every hour! However 250 litres weigh about 500 lb or three times the body-weight of the average man.

Having arrived at this calculation, Harvey at once grasped the absurdity of the assumption that such a volume of blood could constantly seep through the tissue. There was only one way to reconcile these contradictions: the blood which was sent from the heart into the body must return to the heart in order to begin its journey again ... At that moment the idea of a complete circulation of the blood first took root.

Looking back, it seems strange that the idea of a circulatory system of the blood was not arrived at earlier. True, the half-mythical Ancient Chinese emperor, Huang-ti, had hinted at similar trains of thought in his book *Theory of the Interior* (*Nei-Ching*) (see page 42); and the Ancient Indians also seem to have at least sensed the truth about the circulation of the blood. Finally, there are some indications of a similar concept in Hippocrates' writings (see page 75); but even such a great anatomist and dissector as Galen had no idea of the real functions of the heart and blood. In constructing his theories about the movement of the blood he made use of the *spiritus naturalis*, the *spiritus animalis*, and his unshakeable belief in the existence of pores in the dividing wall of the heart (see page 97).

William Harvey was therefore the first man who scientifically proved the existence of the circulatory system. But he was an extremely cautious man. It did not occur to him to publish immediately what he had discovered for he realized what a storm he would arouse when his discovery was made public. While his fame as a doctor grew, he went on dissecting and vivisecting; but however many animals he examined, he never found the pores whose existence had been so stubbornly maintained ever since the days of Aristotle. There could be no doubt about it: the blood must be driven from the left ventricle through the arteries into the body and return via the veins into the right ventricle; from there it must stream into the lungs and from the lungs back into the left ventricle ready to begin the whole process again.

Time and again Harvey confirmed his ideas until at last, in 1628 – in Germany the Thirty Years War had already been raging for ten years – he gave his work *The Movement of the Heart and the Blood* (*Exercitato Anatomica de Motu Cordis et Sanguinis in Animalibus*) for publication to a firm of publishers in Frankfurt. In the preface of this book, which was dedicated to the king of England, in a remarkable mixture of bad Latin and English, Harvey wrote: 'I declare that anatomy cannot be learnt or taught from books or philosophical dogmas, but only in the workshop of nature.'

He then established in sober terms:

. . . that the blood, as a result of the pulsation of the ventricles,
passes through the lungs and the heart and is driven and sent
throughout the whole body, penetrating the veins and the
porosities of the flesh and then, via the veins, from all sides, even
from the periphery to the centre, streaming back from the
little veins into the big ones and from them into the vena
cava, finally reaching the auricle, and in such a great mass,
with such a mighty ebb and flow from here through the
arteries to there, and from there back through the
veins to here, that it cannot be supplied from the nourishment
that has been taken in and moreover in a much greater measure
(than would be possible as a result of the nourishment). It must
therefore be concluded: that in living creatures the blood moves
in a circle by virtue of a certain circular movement and it is
in constant movement and this is the activity of the heart which is
accomplished by means of a pulsation . . .'

What he had feared soon happened. A storm of indignation broke out: people even went so far as to declare Harvey mad. His medical practice suffered heavy losses; but he was able to endure this blow for he was the king's personal physician and, in addition, had wealthy relatives. He was therefore able to go on devoting himself to his studies; they enabled him to recognize that with one stroke, a whole new element had been introduced into the methods of physiological research: weighing and measuring.

The spirit of the times in which Harvey lived also influenced his processes of thought and research; he was less interested in the state of being, than in what happens during this state. It was a time during which the term 'electricity' first appeared; the mystery of the heavens was solved; a time when the thermometer and barometer were invented, when Shakespeare wrote his plays, Rubens, Rembrandt and Van Dyck painted their immortal pictures. Everything was on the move, in a state of flux, and now began a new era for physiology. Now it was no longer a question of learning about the separate parts of the human body; people also wanted to know how everything worked, moved and fitted together. The more descriptive anatomy of previous eras developed into a theory on the function of the organs. The old, often still fantastical, view of nature began to change into experimental research which could not manage without scales and measures; it was, after all, measurements that had provided the flash of inspiration which had helped William Harvey to make his monumental discovery.

When Harvey published his epoch-making work he was fifty years old, but it did not occur to him to rest on his laurels; the many examinations and experiments which he had undertaken to find out the course of the movement of the blood in the body had led his interest in comparative anatomy and embryology to increase more and more. Eagerly, he studied the development of chicks and, once again, he succeeded in making a gigantic step forward – from the point of view of the times he lived in – this time in the field of embryology. At that time there was a widespread belief that, in the embryo, all organs were already fully formed and growth represented merely an enlargement of the embryonic rudiments. Harvey overthrew this generally recognized 'theory of preformation' and instead taught about the gradual building up of the embryo, coining the revealing phrase, *Ex ovo omnia*. He wrote down his experiences in the work *De Generatione Animalum* which was published in 1651.

The more Harvey pursued his scientific studies, the more his practice deteriorated. People also resented his unwavering royalist leanings and his loyalty towards the ill-starred House of Stuart. Even the execution of his monarch, King Charles I, did not make him change his mind; but the fact that that selfsame king, whom he had served as court physician, was forced to mount the scaffold, affected his health as severely as the death of his wife. In addition, he suffered badly from gout which he treated with the most unusual and drastic remedies.

After Charles I's execution Harvey did, in fact, return to London, but his strength was exhausted. He had hardly any patients left, but he was active on behalf of the Royal College of Surgeons for whom he organized a library and a museum. He died in 1657 when he was seventy-nine years old; the influence of his teaching was already apparent during his lifetime. Not only was it recognized that the physiology of the circulatory system had been placed on a totally different basis, but practical medicine also drew practical conclusions from Harvey's theories.

People found out that it was possible to introduce medicines into the body quickly by injecting it into veins and it was realized that, after heavy loss of blood, a transfusion from another person could save people's lives. However, since nothing was yet known about blood groups, there were so many accidents that this procedure was dropped until it came into its own again during the present century with the discovery of the various different types of blood (see page 301). A further result of William Harvey's discovery was a considerable increase in blood-letting.

*The microscope, 'the first great gift which
applied physics passed on to medicine'.
Antonius van Leeuwenhoek, a grocer from
Delft, explored the microcosm and closed the
gap in William Harvey's system of ideas.
Marcello Malpighi, the founder of scientific
microscopic anatomy.*

In spite of his genius, however,
there was one disturbing gap in William Harvey's theories. True,
Harvey had written that the blood in the arteries is sent throughout
the whole body, penetrating the veins and porosities of the flesh
and then, via the veins, even from the periphery to the centre, returns to the heart.' However, since he had no microscope, the
discoverer of the circulatory system could not explain how the
blood, which had been carried throughout the body by the arteries,
reached the veins in order to return to the heart. It was left to
Professor Marcello Malpighi to close this gap. He was an Italian
lecturer at the University of Bologna, and had been born during
that same year, 1628, in which William Harvey's world-shaking
book *De Motu Cordis* was published.

However, before Marcello Malpighi was able to make this
second most significant discovery of the seventeenth century after
William Harvey's, it needed the intervention of a layman to
demonstrate that, by means of the microscope – 'the first great
gift which applied physics passed on to medicine' – it was also

possible to penetrate into the secrets of organisms which, without the help of magnification, could never have been distinguished. The man to whom we owe this intervention was a grocer and cloth merchant, Antonius van Leeuwenhoek, by name. He was born on 24 October 1632 in Delft, south of The Hague, in a house beside one of the little town's many tree-lined canals. He was the off-spring of a line of basketmakers and brewers, and his mother, who had early become a widow, intended him for the civil service.

It may have been a certain restlessness which made him run away from school when he was only sixteen; his next scene of activity was Amsterdam where he was apprentice to a merchant. He stuck that for five years; then he was drawn back to his home town, and after that he began to lead a thoroughly middle-class Dutch existence. He set up as a grocer and cloth merchant and started a family.

Consequently, his life could have taken the same orderly and un-obtrusive course as that of a thousand other of his fellow citizens. Over and above his life as a grocer and head of a family, however, Leeuwenhoek had a strange hobby. For the greatest leisure amuse-ment of this strange, eccentric shopkeeper – who had taken on the job of porter at the local town hall in addition to attending to his shop – consisted of grinding lenses out of fine glass. He had learnt this craft from the opticians, who enjoyed a particularly high reputation in Holland, and now this strange man spent a great deal of his time at his grinding-table, mounting little glass slides in frames made from various different metals, arranging the different lenses in continually varying and carefully tested sequences, in twos or even threes, one after the other, or one above the other, and took pleasure from the fact that the instrument he had con-structed showed objects several times magnified. He constantly went on improving his 'miracle', enlisting the aid of a little concave mirror, which focused the light needed for his intricate examina-tions and – the microscope was born.

It is idle to speculate whether a connection exists between the telescope constructed by Galileo Galilei and the microscope of Antonius van Leeuwenhoek. When the time for a discovery is ripe, it is often made simultaneously in several places, each quite independently of the other. The fact remains that the grocer and porter to the town hall was the first person to use a combination of lenses for exploring the organic world of the microcosm.

Leeuwenhoek's friends and neighbours whispered and made fun of the 'rum fellow' as they called him; but Antonius took no notice. He was in the grip of a craving for knowledge verging on obsession and, as a result, everything which was not securely nailed down had to go under his microscope. Moreover what he saw he neatly wrote down and illustrated with carefully drawn pictures. Scales and hairs, bee-stings and flea-bristles, the proboscis of a gnat and the legs of a beetle, threads of dust and tiny plants found their way under his microscope; he noticed enormous quantities of tiny, moving, multifarious animalcules in a drop of water; and it was also Leeuwenhoek who, among a thousand other things, progressed a good way in the exploration of the micro-scopically small components of human organs. Through his microscope, which showed him a miniature world magnified at most 150 or 200 times, he saw such extraordinary things in human body liquids that he felt dazed at the sight of them.

It is hard to imagine what his sensations may have been as, the first man destined to do so, he gazed into a world which until then had been wholly unknown. One day, when he was examining the transparent tail of a live tadpole through his lenses, he discovered in it an enormous number of very fine blood-vessels which con-nected together the arteries and veins. Thus was the network of hair-fine 'capilliary vessels' discovered and, with it, the picture of the circulatory system outlined by Harvey now had the details filled in.

Leeuwenhoek himself reports thus:

When I examined the tail of this creature, I was presented with a picture which was more beautiful than anything my eyes had seen before. For while the animal lay quietly in the water and I could put it under my microscope just as I liked, I was able to discover fifty blood-circulations in various places. Yet I not only saw how the blood was carried along extraordinarily small vessels from many places in the centre of the tail to the edges, but also that each vessel possessed a curve, or turning-point, which sent the blood back to the centre again, so that it could go on from there to the heart. It now lay open before me that the blood-vessels which I saw in this animal, which are called veins and arteries, are, in fact, one and the same thing; so that inasmuch as they carry the blood to their outermost ends they can rightly be described as arteries; when, on the other hand, they return the blood to the heart, they are veins.

The connection could hardly have been described more clearly. Transported by ingenuous enthusiasm, Leeuwenhoek, with his descriptions, reported everything he had discovered to the Royal Society of Sciences in London.

At first those very learned gentlemen may have raised their eyebrows at the grocer from Delft, but they were clever enough to check his experiments. And, there! Leeuwenhoek had been telling the truth; he had not exaggerated. The rum fellow who, like every true prophet, had so far only been the butt of derision and mockery, was made a member of that learned society and, in gratitude, he reported with redoubled eagerness to the attentive assembly what his microscope had revealed to him.

What Leeuwenhoek unveiled in the world of the miniature was scarcely less important than the discovery of America, and this Columbus of the microcosm succeeded in making more and more discoveries. One day, when he was again studying the network of veins in the transparent tail of a fish, he saw that little oval-shaped bodies were moving along the tubes of the blood-vessels in the blood-liquid. At once he examined some human blood as a comparison: there the little bodies were round. Leeuwenhoek was the first to discover that blood is not an amorphous liquid, but that it is made up of an enormous number of formations called blood corpuscles.

The malice at that time, still permeated with superstition, to which Leeuwenhoek was exposed as a result of his revolutionary discoveries did not cease; but all envy and ill-will rebounded off this stubborn Dutchman and his rock-firm belief in the truth and validity of that which he had found. 'I am absolutely determined', he wrote, 'not just to persist stubbornly in my convictions; I will give them up and be converted to others as soon as sensible, acceptable reasons are given to me to do so. This is the more true since I have no other purpose than to set the truth before my eyes to the best of my strength, to grasp it and to make use of my small talent to free the world of the false doctrines of the ancient heathen, to go over to the truth and to keep fast hold of it.'

No one, however, could dispute the discoveries which Antonius van Leeuwenhoek had made in the microcosm. After a long life spent in pioneering research with his microscope, he died at the age of ninety-one. Whether Marcello Malpighi was in some way influenced by Leeuwenhoek's busy investigations cannot now be determined. However, it was of outstanding importance for further anatomical research with the microscope, that this new branch of science now passed from the hands of this self-taught man into those of a reliable medical scholar; indeed Malpighi can pretty well be regarded as the founder of the science, microscopic anatomy.

Everything which Leeuwenhoek had observed in his ingenuous amateur fashion, now also received scientific confirmation. Malpighi also made experiments on frogs, but he studied the capillary system of the lungs and mesentery of amphibia. Now, at last, the gap was finally closed in William Harvey's theory of the circulatory system, which still existed after Leeuwenhoek's observations. The blood did not ooze away from the split-open ends of the arteries into an 'interdependent river of matter' or 'gaps in the tissue', as Vesalius had supposed, but was taken into a hair-fine vascular system which, penetrating all the regions of the organism, formed a network which transmitted the life-giving fluid to the extremities of the venous system.

That the 'gaps in the tissue' were, however, also involved in a particular way with the 'interdependent river of matter' was established during the seventeenth century by a succession of learned men in Pavia, Padua and Montpellier. They were the first people to describe the lymphatic system which, together with the capillary vessels so important for the processes of life, represented the discovery of yet another element in the flow of body liquid.

Although Malpighi's discovery of the most minute of blood-vessels was important, the further research work of this professor from Bologna was to make him immortal in the realms of medical history. He examined the fine structure of the muscles and bone tissue, the brain, lungs, liver, kidney and spleen, in which he found a great many lymph granules which – like the vascular coils of the kidney – are still known as Malpighian cells today.

Malpighi's method of examining the finer structure of the different organs soon found other adherents and it would be no exaggeration to say that it ushered in a new era in medical history. Descriptions of the different organs were now published in rapid succession and became the signposts for the new way of looking at things; many anatomists who used the new microscope achieved such important discoveries in the course of their research that their names have also come down to posterity as parts of the scientific terminology.

In 1597, Francis Glisson, an English anatomist and professor of medicine from Rampisham in Dorset, wrote a monograph on the liver; in this he described the framework of connective tissue as well as the organ's capsule of connective tissue which is still called Glisson's capsule to this day. He was also the author of the first accurate description of rickets, which was probably the reason why this disease was known abroad as the English illness and not, as many people believe, because it was so prevalent in the slums of the big English towns.

Bauhin's valve, a fold in the mucous membrane between the

small intestine and the colon, was named after Caspar Bauhin, an anatomist, botanist and physician from Basle, who lived from 1560 to 1624. He described this valve in his work *Theatrum Anatomicum* which was published in Frankfurt in 1605 and in which there is also, among other things, the first picture of the suprarenal glands. Another Swiss doctor of the period will also always be commemorated in the history book of medicine: Johann Conrad Peyer, a doctor and anatomist from Schaffhaus who was born in 1653. He discovered a number of lymph follicles in the lower end of the small intestine which are still known as Peyer's patches and which, in cases of diarrhoea and especially typhus, swell up and then can disintegrate to form ulcers.

A third seventeenth century Swiss doctor, who was born in the same year as Peyer, and whose name also lives on in scientific nomenclature, was Johann Conrad Brunner; the small, racemose glands of the duodenum are named after him. In addition to his anatomical discoveries Brunner was an efficient doctor. He acquired many high honours and was appointed physician to the court of the Kurfurst of Pfalz in Mannheim as well as being professor of medicine at the University of Heidelberg.

2 1

Reorganization of scientific thought through Sir Francis Bacon. Physics and Chemistry as the foundations of Iatrophysics and Iatrochemistry. Cartesius regards the living organism as a machine. Santorio and the 'imperceptible body odour'. Borelli solves the mystery of body temperatures. Helmont and the Fermentation. Sylvius extends existing knowledge of the human brain. The rift between the natural sciences and medical science.

T he immense progress in the exploration of the human body and its functions which the seventeenth century brought with it, together with the recent discovery, based on physical considerations, of the circulatory system of the blood, and the development of the telescope invented by Galileo into a microscope, as well as a thousand other things, obviously drew medical science and the natural sciences ever closer together.

Almost half a century earlier, Sir Francis Bacon, Baron Verulam and Viscount St Albans, one-time lord chancellor of England, had announced a reorganization of the sciences or *Instauratio Magna* (the grand instauration). In accordance with this, scientific thought was to be based on methodical discovery and invention, on research and experience. Filled with a deep aversion towards scholastic philosophy, Bacon proclaimed the principle that only independent searching and perception, free of all inherited phantoms, superstitious prejudice and dogma, could form a true picture of the sciences.

Bacon included physics and chemistry in his philosophy of experience; the preservation of health, the healing of disease, and the prolonging of human life he regarded as the chief tasks of medicine. Once again, experience and methodical selection were essential in order to do them justice. The basis was the theory of the construction of the human body and its functions, for which knowledge recourse could also be made to experiments on animals. Systematic records of clinical observations, exact case histories, pathological/anatomical examinations, careful scrutiny of medicines and alleviation of pain were the noblest of the doctor's duties in the cause of a revival of medical science.

It was an immense and forward-looking programme, which Francis Bacon evolved as a result of much constructive thought. Not everything was new; some items had already been introduced, others already anticipated by such people as Roger Bacon (see page 118), Leonardo da Vinci and Paracelsus von Hohenheim (see page 136).

Bacon's warning not to overrate humoral pathology unilaterally and his insistence on the necessity of physical and chemical knowledge, in course of time caused two schools of medicine, based on pure natural science, to come into being. Neither, at first, it is true, produced any noteworthy progress in clinical medicine and both were destined only to have a limited span of life. The new schools were Iatrophysics and Iatrochemistry.

One of the most noted intellects from whom the Iatrophysical school received its stimulus, was the French physician-philosopher René Descartes, latinized into Cartesius, who was born in the Tourraine in 1596. Descartes exercised a lasting influence on contemporary conceptions of the living organism. In drawing the ultimate conclusion from his attempt to explain the phenomenon of life entirely physically by mechanical laws, he arrived at the supposition that the living organism was little more than a brilliant piece of machinery. Queen Christina of Sweden appointed the French philosopher to her court in Stockholm because she had such a high opinion of him and hoped to become better informed as a result of learned conversations with him.

True, even this unusually abstruse thinker also had ideas which seem abstruse to people today. What the Hellenists, Herophilus and Erasistratus (see page 88) had taught about the seat of the soul had sunk into oblivion some time before. For Descartes, the soul was located in the tiny pineal gland, situated in the central cleft of the cerebrum.

Proof of an individual existence, however, was the fact that people think and this produced one of his best-known sayings: 'Cogito ergo sum' – I think, therefore I am. The man who was born eighteen years after William Harvey, and who was to exercise such a far-reaching influence on the whole current of European thought, was not fated to enjoy a long life. He died in Stockholm in 1650 at the age of fifty-four.

No longer was it possible to visualize physiological research without the weighing and measuring; an example of this is in the person of the Paduan and Venetian medical man of letters, Santorio Santorio, who – born in Capodistria, south of Trieste – had a doctor's degree conferred on him when he was only twenty-one. He set himself the special aim of solving the mystery of metabolism which, in the same way as most of the other facts of life, he believed he could trace back to purely physico-mechanical processes. In doing so he reached a dead-end in his speculations from which he could find no way out. He was particularly interested in comparing all that the human body takes in with all that it gives out; and so – apart from the secretions of sweat – he also measured that other imperceptible exhalation on which the ancient physiologists had laid such great weight and which he regarded as highly significant.

Galen had taught that man does not only breathe through his lungs, but that volatile substances can also be exhaled from the body through the skin. In order to understand this *perspiratio insensibilis* accurately, no effort was too much for Santorio. Therefore he built a gigantic weighing machine which was big enough to hold himself, a table and a chair. There he sat, for days and even weeks, measuring exactly what, under all the most varied of living conditions, his body took in and gave off. 'Healthy perspiration is not the secretion of sweat,' he wrote, 'but that hardly noticeable vapour of which about 50 ounces are exhaled every day.'

That would mean 3 lbs in 24 hours! It is needless to say that this calculation far outstrips reality. Like so many an explorer before and after him, Santorio had fallen victim to an error, perhaps because he kept his eye fixed obsessively on the *perspiratio insensibilis* upon which he wanted to base an entirely new theory on sickness and health. Today we know that this 'hardly perceptible body vapour' only amounts to a negligible vaporous exhalation of extracellular fluid.

However Santorio Santorio is not just remembered in medical history for this *perspiratio insensibilis*. It was he who introduced into medical practice a piece of equipment which is still the instrument most commonly used by doctors today: the clinical thermometer. In general, the problems posed by the stability of body temperature in warm-blooded animals was the focal-point of interest among physiologists at that time. Aristotle had taught that the heart was the chief source of body warmth and it was the task of breathing to cool down 'the flame or heat of the heart and supply it with new air'.

One of the first people not content with this explanation which was still widespread even after the circulatory system had been discovered, was the Italian physiologist Giovanni Alfonso Borelli, who lived from 1608 to 1679. Borelli was a member of the learned Accademia del Cimento in Florence, which had been founded by the Medici family. His chief fields of knowledge were mathematics, physics and physiology, and like the other explorers of his time he, too, believed that the facts of life could be fathomed most reliably by experiments and that they operated in accordance with physical and mathematical laws.

Borelli, therefore, also tackled the problem of animal warmth by means of experiments. Like Santorio Santorio, he, too, made use of the thermometer – which had shortly before been invented by his personal friend Galileo – in order to pursue his theories. As animals were not anaesthetized, his experiments seem exceptionally cruel, but they at one stroke served to reduce to absurdity the whole rigmarole of the heart as the source of warmth and the cooling of its 'heat' by the lungs.

Borelli reported the results of his experiment in his book which was published after his death: *De Motu Animalum* (About the movement of the living creature):

In order to find out the exact degree of warmth of the heart, I opened the breast of a living stag in Pisa and immediately inserted a thermometer into the left ventricle of the heart. I found that the highest temperature of the heart did not exceed 40 degrees, that is to say the degree of the sun in summer. After I had measured the temperature of the liver, and the intestines of the same living stag with similar thermometers, I found that both heart and intestines had the same temperature. Therefore the heart cannot be the chief source of animal warmth and it is not necessary for it to be cooled and aired because of its alleged heat. Moreover the cold air does not reach the heart for it is warmed on its way there.

Borelli's exploration had not, it is true, been of benefit to practical medical treatment; physiological research had, however, received an inestimable acquisition. Professor Giorgio Baglivi (1668–1707), who taught in Rome and only lived to the age of thirty-nine, almost went a step further in the physio-mathematical interpretation of the processes of life, especially in the sphere of respiration, glands and the digestive processes. He found parallels between nearly all the organs in the human body and technical instruments such as containers and tubes, scissors and sieves, bottles and bellows, but in the end, Baglivi himself recognized how obscure his approach was. As one extreme often calls up an opposite, he constructed – anticipating later ideas – a mysterious *vis insita*, an inborn power which kept the processes of life going. 'For', as he wrote in his *Praxis Medica*, 'the origin and cause of illness is much too deeply hidden for the human brain to be able to find it.'

Just as the Iatrophysical school produced a whole row of learned men, so, too, did the Iatrochemical one, and their memory also lives on in the history of medicine. The founder, so to speak, of this movement was Johann Baptist van Helmont, who, coming from a noble family in Brabant, was born in Brussels in 1577. He was destined for a medical career, began his studies at Löwen University and soon so distinguished himself there that, at the age of seventeen, he was already giving lectures. Moreover he proved himself a talented all-rounder, for he by no means restricted his studies to medicine, but also devoted himself to astronomy and mathematics, jurisprudence, theology and botany. Later, a wealthy marriage enabled him to make extended educational journeys to Switzerland, Italy, France and England. When he was thirty-two he retired to his country estate in the vicinity of Brussels and from then until he died – persecuted by the Inquisition – at the age of sixty-seven, he lived for his studies.

Van Helmont, who was openly opposed to Galen's humoral pathology, and was an enthusiastic disciple of Paracelsus, added some valuable discoveries to medical science. As a follower of the Iatrochemical school, he held the view that physiological processes were of a chemical nature; it was he who introduced the term 'gases' to describe aeriform substances. He also discovered carbonic acid and recognized that gout was due to an excessive 'acidity' in the blood. Finally, hundreds of years before pepsin was discovered, Helmont put forward the theory that a special substance which combined with gastric acid was involved in the processes of digestion. Since he conjectured that it was also a determining factor in fermentation, he called it *fermentum* and thus, without realizing it, performed an act of baptism which was to have great significance in the future, for in present-day physio-logical chemistry the ferments, or enzymes, play a decisive role. The more research penetrates into the mysteries of living sub-stances, the clearer it becomes that it is always enzymes which direct the processes of life.

Another member of the Iatrochemical school was Franz de Boe who, as was customary at that time, latinized his name to 'Sylvius'. He came from a French Huguenot family called Dubois which had emigrated to Holland and then moved into Germany. Thus Sylvius, who was born in Hanau in 1614, was educated at both a Dutch and a German university. When he was twenty-three years old he received his doctor's degree at Basle and to complete his experience, went to Paris. His path then led him back to the Netherlands where he studied at Leiden University. He agreed with Helmont's view that the transformation of matter in the organism was achieved by fermentation until, as a result of this and the work of the glandular juices, the food had been changed enough to become blood.

Apart from his iatrochemical studies, Sylvius also gave valuable service to the science of anatomy. In Leiden he wrote a book on anatomy in which he extended existing knowledge on the con-struction of the brain in a way that is still valid today. For this, anatomy has awarded him a memorial in scientific nomenclature. The narrow channel running through the cerebellum, connecting the third brain ventricle with the fourth, is still called the *Aquaeductus Sylvii.*

The various different seventeenth century medical systems may have helped theoretical research, but they did not bring much pro-gress to the practical treatment of the sick. An abyss yawned be-tween research and practice. Science and medical treatment no longer seemed to be in harmony. In spite of their basically natural scientific attitudes, several of the guiding principles which Baglivi delivered in his *Praxis Medica*, sound like announcements of bank-ruptcy on behalf of practical medicine. On the other hand, the old Hippocratic medicine, which so many an iatrophysicist and iatrochemist felt was beneath them, was by no means forgotten, as is emphatically revealed by a few further quotations from Baglivi: 'He is a fool who does not read Hippocrates. The past can boast no greater doctor, and the future will not have one. May the doctors at last see sense, wake up out of their deep sleep and recognize how much the virile Ancient Greek medicine differs from the speculative and wavering medical science of today.'

Baglivi's words are eloquent. They reveal the split which existed then between science and practice; they also, however, demonstrated the growing resistance towards Iatrophysics and Iatrochemistry, against a too mechanistic and materialistic conception and interpretation of life and its manifestations. The reaction could not fail to appear. Hippocrates was once more in the ascendant; but the driving force did not emanate – and this is significant – from highly learned university professors, but from a simple London medical practitioner. His name was Thomas Sydenham.

22

*The English Hippocrates, Thomas Sydenham,
who reformed practical medicine and was
the pioneer of a special pathology. The
Dutchman, Herman Boerhaave, who turned
his academy in Leiden into 'the cradle of our
modern clinic'. Albrecht Haller of
Switzerland, the first man in medical history
to write a systematic manual of physiology.*

Thomas Sydenham, who was even in his own days known as 'the English Hippocrates', had an eventful life story. Born in 1624, the son of a distinguished Puritan landowner in Wynford Eagle, Dorsetshire, he joined Cromwell's army during the Civil War. After the Royalists had been beaten he was discharged and, in 1642, at the age of eighteen, he went to study at Oxford, still undecided which discipline to pursue. A doctor called Cox, who was a friend of his, persuaded him to study medicine and in 1648, Sydenham, who, as an ex-soldier in the Parliamentary army, enjoyed special privileges, became a bachelor of arts in medicine.

When Charles II landed in Scotland, Sydenham rejoined the army; he took part in the ensuing war as a captain of cavalry. In 1651 Cromwell defeated Charles II at Worcester; the time had come for Sydenham to return to private life once more. For his services during the war against the Royalists he received a gift of £600. This sum enabled him to establish himself as a doctor in Westminster, south of what was later to be St James's Square.

Only after his military career had come to an end could Sydenham devote all his energy to his medical practice. However, he soon found that, as a result of his years of military service, he had forgotten too much of his medical training. He therefore supplemented his knowledge by further study in Montpellier.

He was thirty-seven years old before he began to practice medicine; it soon became clear, however, that he was taking an entirely different path from that followed by the general medical science of his day. He certainly knew the work of such men as Andreas Vesalius, William Harvey, Marcello Malpighi and Giovanni Alfonso Borelli; but Sydenham did not believe that a practical system of medicine could be built up on the results of such scientific research. He was entirely convinced that no sick man could be cured by learned, scientific-philosophical speculation; as an admirer of Hippocrates and a student of the *Corpus Hippocraticus* (see page 76), he was much more concerned with concentrating on the sick man and his diseases.

Nevertheless, there was a difference between their attitudes. True, Sydenham shared the Hippocratic view that a doctor's chief duty lay in supporting the sick organism in its natural fight against disease. Over and above this, however, the English Hippocrates next directed his attention, in an entirely new way, to the nature of the individual illness. Each illness differed from the next; it was necessary to learn how to distinguish the different illnesses from each other, hence the doctor's work began with diagnosis.

Like Carl Linné, who, during the first half of the eighteenth century, classified all nature's living creatures, so Thomas Sydenham now became the pioneer of a specific pathology. He published excellent descriptions of smallpox, dysentery, scarlet fever, measles and malaria; in fact, infectious diseases were his special interest. Thomas Sydenham was chiefly responsible for establishing quinine, the 'Jesuit's powder' – which had first reached the Old World from the New in 1630 – in the European pharmacopoeia. This is doubly to his credit, showing his lack of prejudice and unbiased judgement, for he remained a staunch Puritan all his life.

His insight into the true and the inorganic diseases was revealed in his book about hysteria. His work on St Vitus's dance was also successful. His description of gout, however, can be called positively classical and probably seems so authentic because Sydenham himself suffered from this disease. 'The victim retires to bed', he wrote, 'and goes to sleep in an entirely healthy condition. At about two in the morning, the sick man wakes up, suffering violent pain in his big toe ... then comes a fit of shivering, followed by a slight fever. The pain increases ... the night is full of anguish ... and an attempt to soften the pain by changing his position is unsuccessful ... the next morning the sick man discovers that his big toe has become swollen ... and a few days' later his other foot starts to throb and swell up.'

Sydenham also made use of blood-letting, which Harvey had made fashionable, though not to such an extent as many of his colleagues. Apart from this, his remedies were simple but effective: against malaria, as already mentioned, he used chinchona rind, against syphilis, mercury; against anaemia, iron. As a faithful disciple of Hippocrates, however, he was constantly at great pains not to disturb the natural healing processes by his medical interventions.

Sydenham's achievements in pioneering a specific pathology soon found adherents; during the following years monographs appeared on many different diseases such as tuberculosis of the lungs and malaria, heart diseases and cerebral haemorrhage, diabetes – now, after thousands of years, it was again observed that the urine of its sufferers had a sweet taste – and hysteria, which at last was identified as a disease of the nervous system and not the uterus ('hysteria' comes from the Greek for uterus); about muscular atrophy and tumours, tropical diseases, forensic medicine and occupational diseases.

Thus the progress that was made in knowledge of different

diseases, no less than practical therapeutics, during the second half of the seventeenth century, compares well with the brilliant results obtained from the anatomical and physiological research undertaken during the first half of that century. Only in surgery were there no comparable advances; in spite of Ambroise Paré's reforms (see page 151), this was still labouring under the effects of its disastrous separation from the rest of medicine. On the other hand, however, thanks to the lead given by the French, the practice of obstetrics registered considerable advances.

The fact that quack remedies and superstition continued to flourish – the French and English kings still undertook to cure sufferers from scrofula by the laying on of hands – had as little power to arrest the progress of medical science as it had in any other age, even the present one.

Thomas Sydenham's work introduced a new era of medical science; and not long afterwards, just as the English Hippocrates had reformed practical medicine, so clinical medicine was also to be revitalized by the work of another great man. It is said that a clinician at Leiden University bared his head every time Sydenham's name was mentioned; the man who showed such deference to the English Hippocrates was Herman Boerhaave, a doctor, who was destined to turn his academy into the forerunner of a modern clinic.

Born in Voorhut near Leiden in 1668, Boerhaave entered the university at the age of fourteen and for the next eight years studied theology, philosophy and mathematics. He took up the study of medicine in 1690 at Leiden, the place which he was later to make the focus of medical science throughout the then civilized world. In 1701, when he was thirty-three, he was already a university lecturer in theoretical medicine; eight years later, when he was a professor, he acquired the chair of botany in addition to that of medicine and, during the winter term, he also gave lectures in chemistry.

Boerhaave's fame as the pacemaker of medical science rests on the fact that he brought classification, cause, nature and treatment of diseases into one clearly arranged system and demonstrated a new approach with regard to clinical education. While he was so engaged, the whole extent of his individual greatness as a doctor and as a person unfolded. He established a hospital expressly for teaching purposes, in which he could combine theoretical and practical instruction at the sick-bed. Here, surrounded by devoted pupils, he demonstrated how to visit patients and taught that, when diagnosing an illness, one should never follow a set dogma but be guided solely by personal observation. By his own example he proved that true care of a doctor for his patients can only stem from a selfless love of humanity.

It was this fundamental reorganization of academic medical instruction which was one of Boerhaave's main achievements. In most universities the clinical instruction of student doctors was exceptionally poor; it was in Leiden that this deficiency was first remedied. In consequence, medical students from all the leading countries flocked to the Dutch university to be taught by the great Boerhaave, whose fame even stretched as far as China.

So, thanks to Boerhaave's reputation, Leiden became the centre of the then medical world, even surpassing time-honoured Padua. Many of Boerhaave's ideas now seem strange – to take only one example, his statement that he had advised an aged burgomaster of Amsterdam to sleep between two young people and that, as a result, the old gentleman had enjoyed visible reanimation, encouragement and access to renewed strength.

Boerhaave was twice nominated rector of Leiden University: in the years 1714 and 1730. When he was forced to resign for the second time – and this time for ever – because of a severe attack of gout, he made his finest and most impressive speech: 'De Honore Medici, Servitute'. (About the honour of being a doctor; readiness to serve). In it he unreservedly testified to Hippocrates' ideas by stating that the doctor must only ever act as the servant of nature and guide its forces into channels which will be helpful to the sick man.

On 23 September 1733, at the age of seventy, the most famous

G 195

doctor of the eighteenth century was released from his grave ill-ness. His remains were laid to rest in the Church of St Peter, Leiden, with all the pomp due to a prince of science; a memorial at Leiden Hospital is a reminder of his fruitful work and the buildings housing the medical faculty were named Boerhaave Kwartier in his honour.

Herman Boerhaave, who could without exaggeration be called the first great clinician in the modern sense of the word, was a rare example of a truly Hippocratic doctor in whom great humanity, goodness, sympathetic understanding and helpfulness, could be combined with learning, perception, knowledge of human nature and intuition. One of his most distinguished pupils wrote of him: 'In scholarship there were some, but not many, who were his equals; but hardly anyone could match his positively saintly character, his kindness towards all people and his benevolence even towards those who envied or opposed him.'

The man who wrote that was Albrecht Haller of Switzerland who, as this example shows, was an ardent devotee of Boerhaave's masterly skill and, at the same time, was himself a talented all-rounder – poet, philosopher, doctor, surgeon, anatomist, physio-logist, botanist, politician and magistrate.

Born in Bern on 16 October 1708 of Swiss upper-class parents, Haller spent the first years of his life on a pleasantly situated country estate, the Hasli-Gut. It was here that the growing boy began to experience that deep, reverent love of nature which was to have such a decisive influence on his entire life and work. When he was thirteen he entered the grammar school in Bern; but only two years later, in 1723, he enrolled in the medical faculty at the University of Tübingen. However, the fairly easy-going life of the Tübingen students did not at all suit the precocious and ambitious young man; in 1725, therefore, only two years later, he moved to Leiden University, attracted by the fame of the great Boerhaave and there, he graduated as a doctor in 1727, when he was nineteen.

His widespread interests, however, and his taste for the encyclopaedic, did no, at first, keep him fixed to one academic discipline; he set off on journeys through various Central European countries; studied higher mathematics at Basle; carried out some practical botany in the Alps and, in 1729, when he was twenty-one, he settled down to practise medicine in his home town, Bern.

He was soon to discover, however, that his fellow countrymen did not have much of a sense of humour: some satirical verses he had published were the cause of his being obliged to wait five years for permission to hold lectures on anatomy at the university. This was not forthcoming until 1734; but neither this, nor his appointments as a doctor to the city and as city librarian, which followed a year later, was enough to satisfy his thirst for scientific activity.

Then, in the spring of 1736, like a ray of light in the darkness, came the call from King George II's minister in Münchhausen, appointing Haller professor of medicine, surgery, anatomy and botany at the newly founded University of Göttingen. Now, when he was twenty-eight, began his heyday. His versatility and his untiring activity brought him triumph after triumph. During his years at Göttingen, Haller set up an anatomical institute, laid out a botanical garden, founded a journal, the *Götting Journal of Learned Matters*, started a maternity clinic and established the Royal Society of Sciences, of which he was granted the life-long presidency. Honours and distinctions for the world-famous scholar poured in from all the civilized countries. Emperor Francis I raised him to the nobility.

Meanwhile Haller untiringly continued to pursue his scientific activities. He published an atlas on the anatomy of blood-vessels, which contained model copperplate illustrations. In doing so, he again discovered something new – he clarified the intricate connections of the portal venous system; and science has rewarded him by perpetuating his name in the concept *Tripps Halleri* – in scientific nomenclature.

However, it was particularly his achievements in the realms of physiology which really made him the great pioneer of medicine and anthropology that he was. He tried to draw into one system the results of the diverse and revolutionary anatomical and physio-logical research of the past decades which then were still uncon-nected, each standing separately on its own. To do this, he chiefly made use of experimental physiology and the systematic examina-tion of the activities of the different organs. In place of the purely mechanical and chemical conception of the vital functions, then still considered valid, he put the knowledge that muscles and nerves each have specific biological qualities peculiar to them-selves. He taught that 'excitability' or 'irritability' was charac-teristic of the muscular tissue, whereas for the nerves it was the sensitive faculty or 'sensibility'. Muscular contractions and nerve impulses were accordingly 'vital functions' which could not be explained by either chemical or physical laws.

Haller collected all the results of the research which he had undertaken, together with the knowledge gained from experience and experiment, into the first systematic manual of physiology in medical history: *Primae Lineae Physiologiae* (Ground-lines of physiology). It was later followed by an extensive eight-volume handbook of anatomy and embryology entitled *Elementa Physio-logiae Corporis Humani*, a monumental work that assured its author a lasting place of honour among those who advance the cause of medicine, in spite of the fact that it exhibits certain deficiencies which to us now seem surprising. In spite of the funda-mental discoveries of Leeuwenhoek and Malpighi, Haller was of the opinion that working with a microscope was an entirely useless activity; he still held fast to the old mistaken view that animal warmth was caused by a process of friction in the blood. As a 'preformist' he also firmly believed that man was preformed in miniature in the germ-cell; and in his *Elementa* appears the following sentence: 'There is no change; no part of the body is made before another; all are created at once.'

The man who was destined to correct this particular mistake was Karl Friedrich Wolff. Throughout more than ten years of extensive correspondence, he tried to argue Haller out of his mistaken ideas – but in vain. The great man from Switzerland resisted the idea that a man gradually developed from quite simple basic beginnings into his final form. Albrecht Haller's attitude was an example of the split in the baroque mode of thought; in spite of the rationalism which controlled his scientific and medical reasoning, as a practising Christian he was not prepared to make any concessions.

We do not know what caused the great professor – who meanwhile had also been appointed a member of the grand council of his native city – in 1753 when he was forty-five and at the height of his fame, suddenly to give up all his offices and return to his home in Switzerland. His scientific work, however, continued unceasingly even in Bern where, after his return, he was given an appointment as city magistrate.

During the following years he kept in touch with Göttingen, the place where he had done his most successful work, as well as with other scientific centres of the world. Moreover his activities generally continued to be varied: he managed the saltworks in Bex and Aigle, founded an orphanage in his home town, busied himself in politics and technical administration and wrote political novels – to mention only a few of them.

It is quite obvious that a flame which is so fierce must burn itself out before its time. Haller went to his rest when he was only sixty-five, the victim of continual illnesses and depressions; and on 12 December 1777 his brilliant flame of life was extinguished for ever.

23

*The dispute about the embryonic theory.
The discovery of spermatozoa and graafian
follicles. The theory of preformation. Karl
Friedrich Wolff's pioneering work: 'Theoria
Generationis' brings about the collapse of the
theory of preformation. Karl Ernst von Baer
discovers the human egg.*

As mentioned briefly in the preceding chapter, one of the advocates of medical science to whom Albrecht Haller was most violently opposed was Karl Friedrich Wolff, the 'learned doctor of medicine'. In order to see just how much he achieved in advancing the knowledge of physiology and anthropology, it is necessary to go back a little in time. In the seventeenth and eighteenth centuries all learned men, without exception, were still gripped by the unshakable conviction that the human embryo was nothing other than a complete human being in minute form; that is to say, a miniature adult human being. All the parts of the body, such as organs, etc., were already present from the moment when the development began, completely formed in advance, albeit in a much smaller form.

This concept, which was called the theory of preformation, still survived even after the invention of the microscope, although no one succeeded in discovering in the ovum the supposedly complete parts of the body. Therefore it was supposed that, at the earliest stages of development, all these 'preformed' parts, such as bones, nerves, blood-vessels, etc., were still completely transparent and that was why it was not possible to see them; they only lost their transparency as they increased in size. As they grew bigger, the parts revealed themselves like a plant-bud burgeoning into blossom. The German word for development – literally, unwinding – still reflects this idea. If anyone expressed the opinion that there might be organs which were not yet present in the ovum, then such a theory came under violent attack.

One of Antonius van Leeuwenhoek's pupils, a student named Hamm, who came from Leiden, was the first person to see a mass of tiny, fast-moving, threadlike structures in the live seminal fluid. The diligent Leeuwenhoek at once seized upon this discovery and caused a sensation with its publication.

Also living in Delft, at the same time as Leeuwenhoek, was the Dutch anatomist, Regnier de Graaf. De Graaf, who was nine years younger than Leeuwenhoek, had studied medicine in Löwen, Utrecht and Leiden, and, as a result of his services to research on the female ovaries, became a corresponding member of the Royal Society in London; it was he who had first put the amateur microscopist in touch with that learned society. The worthy doctor, who died in 1673 when he was only thirty-two, discovered strange, blisterlike growths in the female ovary, five millimetres in diameter, which, in those days, were thought to be the human eggs and which are still to this day known as Graafian follicles.

Now that the two elements necessary for germination had been discovered and it was known that they had to meet in order to permit the formation of a new human being, the preformists were clearly in an awkward situation. Was the preformed human being to be found in the egg or the spermatozoan? Leeuwenhoek was of the opinion that the future human was preformed in the sperm cell which his pupil had discovered and that the ovum served as nourishment to it. Other scientists maintained that the miniature human was preformed in the ovum and at once the 'animalculists' and 'ovists' confronted each other in fierce controversy. True, the number of 'animalculists' was the greater; they even went so far as to depict the little human with his body curled round, his knees drawn up and hands pressed against the enormous head in the top or 'head' end of the spermatozoan, as did the Dutchman Hartsoeker towards the end of the seventeenth century.

However, the real function of the sperm cell, it is true, still remained shrouded in obscurity for a long time to come, although the Italian, Lazzaro Spallanzani proved, during experiments made by filtering animals' semen, that it was the sperm bodies and not the seminal fluid as such which were concerned in fertilization.

Distinguished physiologists debated in all seriousness whether the sperm cells ought to be regarded as parasitic forms of life or as 'the primitive living part of the animal in which they are to be found'. The possibility was therefore left open that the sperm cell might live inside the human body as independent infusoria; but this theory was destroyed by an anatomist and physiologist named Kölliker, who was born in Würzburg in 1817, and who produced proof that the spermatozoa were produced by special cells in the male generative gland.

The preformation theory, of course, received its death-blow when a histology of cells was established; but even before this it had been exposed by Karl Friedrich Woff who, as a result of his life's work, is regarded as the founder of modern embryology. This pioneer of embryology was to enjoy a strange destiny. Born in Berlin in 1733, he studied natural science and medicine in that town and in Halle; when he was twenty-six he startled the world by publishing a doctor's thesis which was at once the most famous, the most sensational and the most influential work of his life.

The title of this thesis was *Theoria Generationis*. It appeared in 1759 and was to introduce a new era in embryology, and in its reference to the histology of cells, was actually eighty years ahead of its time. In it, Karl Friedrich Wolff explained that the assumption according to which the embryo was, so to speak, a miniature edition of the finished creature with all its organs existing or 'preformed' on a tiny scale, was false. Supporting his argument with careful observations, he proved that the embryo is primarily a simple structure, as yet containing no organs, and that as a result of a progressive development the simple structure becomes a complex organism ready for birth.

The reverberations caused by Wolff's *Theoria Generationis* were phenomenal. The young candidate for a doctor's degree was violently attacked by almost all the learned men of science; the saying coined by the physicist and satirist from Göttinger Georg Christoph Lichtenberg, a contemporary of Karl Friedrich Wolff, seems apt: 'It is almost impossible to carry the torch of truth through a crowd without singeing someone's beard'.

The loudest voice raised against Karl Friedrich Wolff was, as mentioned before, that of Albrecht Haller. How considerable was his public influence and that of the other preformists is illustrated with frightening clarity by the fact that Wolff's request to hold lectures in physiology was refused.

Therefore he took part in the Seven Years' War as a military doctor and looked after the sick and wounded in the Silesian military hospitals. After the peace treaty was signed at Hubertusberg, Karl Friedrich Wolff waited another three years for his appointment as a university lecturer – in vain; it continued to be stubbornly withheld from him. All too tragically the saying about a prophet counting for nothing in his own country was in his case again proved true. However, foreign countries were more perceptive. In 1766 Empress Catherine of Russia appointed him to the Academy of St Petersburg and he was destined to enjoy almost thirty years of fruitful work before he died in the Russian capital in 1794.

So Kaspar Friedrich Wolff was not, himself, destined to experience the clear and unequivocal confirmation of his discovery – the histology of cells. For with this discovery, that is to say with the establishment of the fact that the cell is the foundation stone of every living thing, the preformation theory collapsed like a house of cards. With the knowledge that the human being is composed of a vast number of cells and that each new human is created by constant divisions taking place in one cell – the fertilized ovum – the assumption that all parts of an organism exist in a minute form in the embryo had lost all sense.

The human ovum also was discovered, sixty-eight years after Karl Friedrich Wolff's pioneering work *Theoria Generationis* had appeared.

For one-and-a-half centuries, since the days of Regnier de Graaf, people had thought they knew the human ovum; but what was believed to be the ovum – the Graafian follicle, five millimetres in size – proved only to be the container; the real egg cell measuring only seventeen hundredths of a millimetre, lay surrounded by fluid inside the Graafian follicle.

Just twelve years before Theodor Schwann established his histology of cells, the man who was to see the first real human ovum was an Estonian, one of the most widely respected and brilliant men of science of his era – Karl Ernst von Baer by name. He was born in 1792 on his parents' country estate in Estonia, studied medicine in Dorpat and then travelled to Würzburg in Germany where he studied comparative anatomy. In 1818 he was appointed professor of zoology in Königsberg; in 1862 he took over the direction of the Anatomical Institute there and a year later he succeeded in making his great discovery: the human ovum. He published his conclusions the same year in a work: *De Ovi Mammalium et Hominis Genesi* (About the formation of the egg in mammals and humans).

Karl Ernst von Baer was also given an appointment in St Petersburg. He spent many years doing various kinds of research at the St Petersburg Academy and making several voyages of discovery until in 1876, when he was eighty-four, he died in Dorpat.

24

Maria Theresa appoints Gerard von Swieten
of Leiden as her personal physician in
Vienna. The old-fashioned Viennese medical
faculty. Anton de Haen extends
the clinical system. Foundation of the
Royal Academy of Surgery in France. In
England, John Hunter pioneers scientific
pathological anatomy. Giovanni Battista
Morgnani breaks new ground with his
'The Seat and Causes of Diseases', *the first*
handbook of the new pathological anatomy.
Auenbrugger initiates the practice of
'percussion'.

Albrecht Haller's world-wide
reputation as a man of learning and one of the best-known
scientists of his day was so great that an amusing anecdote circulated about him. A pirate, who was busy plundering a ship,
came across a box which bore on its lid the inscription: 'Books
for Professor Albrecht von Haller'. The pirate so admired the
Swiss doctor's genius that he left the box untouched.

Meanwhile, Haller was not the only one of the great Boerhaave's pupils to achieve honour and fame. A man who was no
less energetic and successful followed in Boerhaave's footsteps.
By a strange sequence of political events, it was to be his destiny
to remould the medical faculty and, especially, the clinic in distant

Vienna, in accordance with Boerhaave's ideas. Gerard von Swieten, this favourite pupil of the great man, was born in Leiden in 1700 where he received his doctor's degree at the age of twenty-five.

At that time the medical faculty in the Austrian capital was in a sorry plight. When Maria Theresa began her reign in 1740, she recognized with characteristic farsightedness that a thorough reform of university education was urgently needed.

As chance would have it, the Archduchess Maria Anna, Maria Theresa's heavily pregnant sister, lay seriously ill in Brussels at that time, and neither Maria Theresa's personal physician, Engels, nor the other doctors in Brussels who were called in, were able to help. The court therefore decided to consult a doctor at the famous Leiden clinic and the choice fell on Gerard von Swieten. His demeanour impressed her so greatly that without hesitation, in a warm-hearted personal letter which still is in existence, she appointed the forty-five-year-old doctor to be her personal physician in Vienna.

It was not an easy decision for Gerard von Swieten to make. However, the fact that as a Catholic he would never be awarded a professorship in Leiden and, therefore, could never become Boerhaave's successor, proved decisive. So, in the summer of 1745, von Swieten moved to Vienna; and it was soon to prove that, with his outstanding talent for organization, he was the right man in the right place. Under von Swieten's direction and with Maria Theresa's sympathetic support, not only the medical faculty but the entire Austrian medical practice was fundamentally reorganized, and von Swieten was himself appointed director and president of the medical faculty by imperial patent.

A passage that he wrote about the clinical tuition he administered is characteristic of von Swieten's systematic procedure:

During the space of two years I shall lecture about medicine
and display the functions of the human body, its physiology
– that is, I shall seek to make clear to my listeners the structure

of our bodies by means of anatomical specimens which, at much trouble and great expense, I have collected for my own instruction and also for that of my children, should I discover in them a desire and love for medical science . . . During the second year I shall deal with pathology, that is the theory of diseases, their causes, characteristics and symptoms as well as remedies and their application. Thus I shall arrive at the *materia medica*, that is, the drugs, their dosage, their preparation, etc . . .

Gerard von Swieten, through his revival of the Viennese medical school, gave Europe a 'new medical focus'; in his old age he completed the *Commentaries to Boerhaave's Aphorisms* which soon became an almost indispensable handbook for medical men. Before he died, on 18 June 1772, he had, in his selfless way, provided a suitable successor. In 1754 he had called to Vienna Anton de Haen who was another of Boerhaave's pupils. Haen, who was head of the clinic, was born in The Hague in 1704; believing that experience and tuition at the sick-bed were more important than anything else to the progress of medicine he expanded still further the clinical system which Boerhaave had created, and set down his vast number of observations, clinical pictures and case histories in his eight-volume work, *Ratio medendi* (The law of healing).

After the remarkable progress made by clinical medicine during the eighteenth century, it was obvious that surgery would now advance to take its rightful place in the scientific structure of medicine. France began the progress; again, a chance event was the cause. The 'sun king' Louis XIV, was suffering from a fistula in the anus, of which tiresome complaint he was cured by surgical intervention. As a result, the French surgeons acquired a high reputation; the foundation of the Royal Academy of Surgery, which only took place after Louis's death, brought full recognition to the surgical profession in France.

However, across the channel, surgery was also about to make

significant advances. These are especially associated with the name of a Scot called John Hunter who was born in 1728, studied medicine at Oxford and, after working for a time as a surgeon, took part in various military campaigns as a staff-surgeon. Hunter was a strange man and full of ideas. His interests were by no means confined to surgery, he also studied every aspect of nature with passionate curiosity and concern, and was an inveterate collector. 'When I was a boy,' Hunter wrote of himself, 'I wanted to find out all about clouds and grasses, and why the leaves change their colour in the autumn. I watched the ants, the bees, the birds, the tadpoles and grubs . . .'

In Hunter there was still something of the all-round genius of earlier days; he did not just transform surgery from a craft into a branch of science; he worked out important conclusions about the processes of inflammation, suppuration and regeneration; founded scientific dentistry and became a pioneer in comparative and pathological anatomy.

With Edward Jenner, one of the most famous doctors in medical history, of whom mention will be made later, he studied the phenomenon of the stability of body heat, as well as that of hibernation. As a result of what Hunter found out about the temperature of hibernating animals, he imaginatively put forward the idea, which kept reappearing, but which is today recognized as impracticable, that the limit of a lifespan could be interrupted by slowly freezing people and then allowing them to thaw out again centuries later. In 1775, John Hunter reported to the Royal Society about the unvarying temperature in healthy people and, since then, the stability of body heat has been a scientific fact.

A thorough examination of John Hunter's life suggests that, in the end, his medico-surgical activities were not his prime concern. In spite of the fact that, as a highly respected surgeon, he could command high fees, he was constantly in debt, for his real hobby was collecting animals. In order to indulge in this hobby to his heart's content, he bought a large estate with a country house and park, where he kept numerous mammals, birds and fishes. In another great building in Leicester Square, London, he, who was the real founder of all natural history collections, displayed some 13,600 specimens illustrating human and comparative anatomy, as well as pathology – and among them some most remarkable curiosities. After Hunter's death, the collection was bought by the British government for £15,000; it can still be seen in the Royal College of Surgeons where it fills no less than five rooms.

The last part of John Hunter's life was overshadowed by illness. The indefatigable, ever-curious man was eager to find out whether in fact – as was assumed at that time – syphilis and gonorrhoea were one and the same disease. He therefore inoculated himself with the pus of a patient who was, unfortunately, suffering from both diseases at the same time. The consequence of this brave experiment on himself was that Hunter contracted both syphilis and gonorrhoea. Both were in the highest degree dangerous to him, for he was in any case already suffering from angina pectoris; and so, in 1793, when he was only sixty-five years old, he went to his final rest.

Progress in pathology was not just confined to Northern Europe; about the same time as Hunter was helping to bring about a break-through in scientific pathological anatomy in Great Britain, in 1761 a revolutionary work appeared in far-off Italy, which bore the title, *The Seat and Cause of Disease*. By publishing this monumental work, the author, Giovanni Battista Morgnani, gave the lie to all those who maintained that after a certain age the human mind must begin to lose its keenness. When he published his life's work, which was based on more than seven hundred post-mortem examinations, he was seventy-nine years old!

Morgnani was born in a house in Forli, in the then Papal States; there Giovanni Battista first saw the light of day in 1682. He studied medicine in Bologna and already displayed his unusual scientific talent by acting for a year as substitute for his teacher, the famous anatomist Valsalva, whose name lives on in 'Valsalva's experiment' – the experiment to prove the existence of a passage through the eustachian tube. After he had ended his studies, however, he bade farewell to research for the time being and settled down as a doctor in his home town.

However, once he had enjoyed such a lively contact with scientific research, the daily routine of a doctor's practice could not satisfy him for long. Therefore he regarded it as a deliverance when, in 1711, at the age of twenty-nine he was appointed professor of theoretical medicine, and shortly afterwards also of anatomy, at the famous University of Padua, so rich in traditions.

Now commenced an extremely productive period for Morgnani. He began a work which was to occupy him for half a century. He observed the appearance of various diseases, made dissections and experiments on animals and tried to make use of what he found to explain the clinical picture. He was no longer merely concerned with the anatomy of the healthy organism which had already been so widely explored; he was investigating the origin and seat of diseases which produce changes in the various organs; all that he discovered during years of laborious work he arranged, from the head to the feet, in a grand exhaustive system. The result was his five-volume work, mentioned earlier, *De Sedibus et Causis Morborum*, which has justly been described as 'the first handbook of the new anatomical pathology'. This pioneering work has earned Morgnani a lasting place among the really great names of medical science.

He still had ten years to live before dying on 6 December 1771 when he was almost ninety. His name is not only linked to the great work which had introduced a whole new epoch in medical science, but is also perpetuated in the description of various organs and symptoms of disease of the human being.

With Giovanni Battista Morgnani, who was the first person to make a systematic examination of the connection between symptoms of disease and post-mortem results, pathology began to acquire an anatomical orientation in that it was increasingly realized that anatomical changes in the organs or body systems are imprinted on the clinical picture. From this recognition, it was only a step to the desire to find some way of discovering possible anatomical abnormalities in living bodies, and so find a solution to the disease.

A doctor of the Viennese school, called Leopold Auenbrugger, blazed a trail in this direction. He was born in 1722, the son of a publican, and from his boyhood had observed his father rapping the casks with his knuckles in order to find out the level of the contents by the sound of the knock. Later on, after Auenbrugger had studied medicine under Gerard von Swieten and become a doctor, he remembered his boyhood experiences and developed a way of finding out the condition of the organs inside by listening to the echo produced by knocking on the patient's thorax.

For seven years Auenbrugger worked at his 'percussion' procedure, publishing his findings during the same year that the elderly Giovanni Battista Morgnani brought out his book about the seat and origin of disease. Auenbrugger's book, *Inventum Novum* – in which, as in Morgnani's work, an attempt was made to find a method of discovering local symptoms of disease – in spite of introducing a new era in the field of physical diagnosis found little recognition during the author's lifetime. It was not until half a century later that the significance of Auenbrugger's method was recognized and brought into general use (see page 256).

25

*The Englishman, Priestley, and Scheele,
the chemist from Stralsund, discover
oxygen. The Frenchman, Lavoisier, explains
the mystery of respiration and recognizes
life as a process of combustion. The Italian,
Spallanzani, refutes the error or mistaken
idea of 'spontaneous generation'. Claude
Bernard of France founds modern
experimental physiology.*

While immense advances were being made in clinical medicine, surgery and anatomical pathology, physiological research did not stand still; in addition, physics and chemistry became more and more indispensable auxiliaries of medical science. Revolutionary findings were made particularly in the fields of respiration and metabolism. Already during the second half of the seventeenth century, the English naturalist, Robert Boyle, had perceived the chemical nature of air, and thus the possibility of a gaseous form of matter. About a century later, his fellow countryman, Joseph Priestley – theologian, philosopher, chemist and physicist – discovered the gas, oxygen. Leonardo da Vinci had already established, three centuries earlier, that there were two components in atmospherical air: one which supported respiration and combustion and another which did not.

Priestley, who was born in 1733 in Fieldhead, near Leeds, in the county of Yorkshire, was an extraordinarily versatile man.

He was employed at different times as a preacher, a professor of literature and a librarian; in 1780 he became the minister of a Birmingham congregation composed of all dissenting noncomformist protestants outside the established Church. However, because of his liberal ideas, the 'orthodox' ministers managed to rouse the people against him to such an extent that in 1791 – the same year that across the Channel in Revolutionary France, the legislating assembly ordered the deportation of all priests who refused to take an oath – they destroyed both his church and his home. No alternative was left for this otherwise fearless man but to flee to Pennsylvania in the USA, where he became the founder of the Unitarian Church.

In 1774, when Priestley was still employed as librarian to Lord Shelburne, he discovered oxygen and recognized its indispensability and vital necessity to man and beast. Since it was 'in the air' at that time, a chemist from Stralsund called Scheele made the same discovery independent of Priestley and christened oxygen 'fire-air'. At first the gas was also called 'life-air', understandably so, as it is this component of the atmosphere which supports respiration and combustion in human beings; indeed, man and beast only breathe in order to extract the life-giving gas, or oxygen from the air. Plants, however, as Priestley observed, are able to 'refresh' the air that has had its oxygen content used up to such an extent that it can once again serve for respiration and combustion.

The scientists who were struggling to discover the secrets of the human organism, had now come close to finding out the connection between respiration and the circulation of the blood, and the metabolic nature of what is called life! Only one tiny step separated them from the knowledge that life represents a process of combustion which is not possible without oxygen.

The man who took this last step was a French chemist from Paris called Antoine Laurent Lavoisier, an extremely discerning observer, who studied law and natural science and, when he was only twenty-five, entered the French Academy of Sciences. Indefatigably, he conducted experiments and, as a result of his brilliantly conceived tests, he confirmed that when inhaling the organism takes oxygen from the surrounding air in order to maintain the combustion process, which can also be called the action of living; and that when breathing out, the waste products of the fires of life – carbon dioxide and water – are eliminated.

The end of this distinguished man was tragic. He was a victim of the French Revolution. Since he was one of the general tax-collectors, the tribunal of the Terror were provided with an easy pretext for a denunciation. On 8 May 1794 the executioner's assistant led him to the guillotine. It had been fruitless to point out to the tribunal his great services to medicine. 'The Republic needs no learned men,' came the reply. 'Justice must take its course.' When Lavoisier mounted the scaffold, the mathematician Lagrange murmured to astronomer Delambre– to have said it aloud would have been dangerous – 'One moment suffices to strike off his head; but perhaps a hundred years will pass before we shall see another man of his stature.' He was to be proved right.

No less revolutionary than the discoveries in the field of respiration were those which were revealed during experiments to explain the processes of metabolism. Galen's old theory, according to which the eaten food is turned into blood in the liver (see page 97), no longer satisfied anyone; one of the first people who undertook to refute this idea was Lazzaro Spallanzani – the Italian physicist and physiologist of whom mention has already been made. The Swiss medical historian, Erwin H. Ackerknecht, described him as 'one of the most remarkable scientists of all time' and this opinion is no exaggeration for Spallanzani was a remarkably original thinker, interested in a variety of subjects, fond of travelling, bubbling over with ideas, and always ready to make new discoveries. He was born in Scandiano not far from Modena, about a century after Harvey had made known his discovery. His father, who was a lawyer, intended that his son should also follow the law.

When he was still only a boy, however, Lazzaro was already filled with such an obsessive urge to unravel the mysteries of nature that in the end his father gave him permission to study natural science at the University of Reggio in Emilia. Spallanzani was not yet thirty when – in addition to his study of mathematics and literature, publishing translations of classical poetry and becoming ordained as a priest – he was appointed a professor of Reggio University; soon his fame had spread to all the centres of learning in Europe. He took part in an extensive correspondence with Frederick the Great, who made him a member of the Prussian Academy of Sciences in Berlin, and Frederick's great antagonist, Maria Theresa, appointed him professor of natural science at the University of the then Austrian town of Pavia, where he was also to become head of the Museum of Natural History.

Spallanzani is known in scientific circles as being one of the most prolific contributors to the development of medical science. He lives on in the opera, *Tales of Hoffmann*, the first act of which is based on E. T. A. Hoffmann's story *The Sandman* from the book *Night Pieces*. In this, he figures as a cynical physicist who, with Coppelius, the mechanic, constructs the mechanical doll, Olympia.

This negative characterization of the great natural scientist, who had brought a new spirit of life into the University of Pavia which had fallen into a kind of Sleeping Beauty trance, may have been the result of the intrigues of his colleagues to which the professor was exposed. His co-professors were furious because their lecture rooms remained almost empty whereas, during one of Spallanzani's lectures, there was scarcely enough room to contain his audiences.

While Spallanzani was away on one of his many journeys to Germany, Switzerland, the East and the Mediterranean, a trap was secretly being set for him at home, which it was intended should finish him once and for all. In his home town, Scandiano, he had set up a small private collection of natural science exhibits and now, some of those who envied him, had sent a spy to his private museum and there found labels belonging to the museum of the University of Pavia. At once Spallanzani was accused of theft and defamed in the most unspeakable manner. His students, however, loyally stood by him and the imperial government in Vienna not only rehabilitated him magnificently but, without further ado, threw his detractors out of the university.

Spallanzani's greatest service, however, was to demonstrate once and for all, by means of irrefutable practical experiments, the absurdity of the erroneous theory of 'spontaneous generation' of living creatures from inanimate substances. In addition, he was keenly interested in discovering how the human body transforms the food it eats into bodily materials for the support of life and also for the replacement and renewal of used-up and worn-out parts.

Spallanzani, too, had long ceased to believe in Galen's theory on the constant transformation of food into blood in the liver. He felt certain that this mysterious process of transformation began in the stomach. So he tried to solve the mystery by performing rigorous experiments on himself. He carved himself some little wooden tubes with openings in their sides. Then he slipped pieces of meat into the hollow spaces in the tubes and swallowed them. After a while, he poked a finger into his throat and vomited up the wooden tubes in order to see how the pieces of meat had changed as a result of their sojourn in his stomach.

As a result of these drastic experiments, he succeeded in making a number of highly significant discoveries which he only stopped when an uncontrollable nausea prevented him from continuing. He managed to dispel the erroneous belief, widespread at that time, that the transformation of food in the stomach was based on a process of decomposition. Almost more important still to the study of human physiology was the discovery that the lining of the stomach secretes a specific gastric juice which is indispensable to the start of the digestive process. Spallanzani was able to curdle milk with this juice and it seems almost incredible that such a clever man should not have drawn the obvious conclusion that the gastric juice must contain an acid ...

Spallanzani died in 1799; however, the problem of metabolism continued to preoccupy the followers of medical and physiological science. True, it was once again a question of a collision of hostile views, but again progress was born of this conflict. A Frenchman, Theophile Bordeu – born in 1722 – was a lecturer at the revered University of Montpellier; he represented most clearly the opposition to the assumption that the processes of life could be explained by means of anatomical, chemical and physiological data. Instead, he believed that a special 'life force', a *vis vitalis*, gave organisms of the higher orders the ability to exist and support those processes which could, taken together, be described as life.

As a result of a firm belief in the existence of this life force, the conviction prevailed that it would never be possible to manufacture organic substances from chemical elements. This dogma was shattered when, in 1828, a few decades later, the Göttinger research scientist Friedrich Wöhler, succeeded in producing urea artificially, a distinct product of animal metabolism, from its individual chemical constituents, in his retort, and quite without any mysterious 'life force'.

A great event often brings others in its train; Wöhler's achievement was the green light for a new phase of research into the processes of metabolism in living organisms. Research scientists were looking for the striking chemical changes which an organism must regularly and continuously make in order to turn the components of food into those substances necessary to sustain life.

Once more the strange phenomenon occurred; in countries which were geographically far apart, different scientists were searching for the same things entirely independent of each other. In Germany it was the research scientists, Friedrich Tiedemann and Leopold Gmelin, whose names will eternally be associated with the history of medicine. Born in 1781, Tiedemann had been working since 1816 as professor of zoology, anatomy and physiology in the University of Heidelberg where he built the anatomical theatre. Gmelin, born in 1788, the offspring of an old, well-known, professorial family in Göttingen, was also at Heidelberg as professor of medicine and chemistry. Thus the fields of interest of the two scientists were complementary to each other and to their collaboration science owes the first comprehensive and really successful treatment of the whole theory of metabolism.

As early as 1820 the two scientists published a work entitled *Experiments on the ways in which substances from the stomach and intestinal canal reach the blood.* This small work contained knowledge which, for that time, can be described without exaggeration as epoch-making. It explains the significance of the lymphatic system in the absorption of certain components of food, the spleen is described as a blood-forming organ and the fallacious belief in the existence of 'secret urinary passages' which had stubbornly persisted until then, was exploded once and for all.

The further co-operation of the two learned men – a fruitful synthesis of anatomical, chemical and microscopic methods of examination, as well as physiological experiments – helped to produce a further work entitled *Experiments on Digestion*, which was written only a few years later and, in 1824, entered as a prize essay in the competition organized by the French Academy of Sciences. The judges, however, lacked the necessary perception to recognize the lasting significance of this basic work; they merely bestowed on it an 'honourable mention'. This was, however, politely declined by the two authors, so the work *Experiments on Digestion* was brought out in 1826-7 by a German publisher.

In this uncommonly painstaking work, based on practical experience, the problems of metabolism were seen in sharper outline. The two professors from Heidelberg stated that the food is dissolved by the saliva in the mouth with the gastric juices and gastric movements continuing this process; and both depend to a great extent on the amount and 'digestibility' of the food eaten. Hydrochloric acid was recognized as an active ingredient of the gastric juice, the chemical composition of the bile was described and its significance in the digestive process explained, and the characteristics of the bile pigments examined.

As was only to be expected, Tiedemann's and Gmelin's work acted as the prelude to a great number of other dissertations and experiments undertaken in different institutes and laboratories to discover more about the manifold processes of metabolism. In the New World an American army surgeon called William Beaumont had a stroke of luck during one of his examinations. He had an opportunity to study in a living patient the way in which a sojourn in the intestines, and in particular the effect of the gastric juice, changes the food which has been eaten. A Canadian hunter named Saint-Martin was suffering from a rifle shot which penetrated the stomach wall; even though the wound itself healed, a fistula remained through which the gastric juice constantly dripped.

Beaumont then hit on an idea which in those times was very daring: artificially to introduce food into the stomach of this human 'guinea pig', to withdraw it again after a time by the same route and then to examine it to see what effect the gastric juices had had on the food.

To this end he put small morsels of various foods into little gauze bags and, via the fistula, placed them in the Canadian's stomach. After a certain time the gauze bags were withdrawn and then examined at leisure in the laboratory to see what changes had taken place in the food.

From this instructive process it was only a step to the introduction of artificial stomach fistulas in suitable animals for experiment, and it was thanks to such experiments that in the days to come, many more discoveries were made in the field of metabolism.

Claude Bernard, who was born in 1813, the son of a Burgundian wine-grower, was a research scientist who made a special study of such experiments. It was he who laid the foundation of the whole great structure of modern experimental physiology. Almost all his contemporaries were still haunted by a belief in the existence of 'life force'. However, Bernard was much too sceptical a man to believe in any mysterious force or combination of forces which could direct and regulate an organism. Such a concept was not in keeping with his scientific way of thinking; he felt certain that any organism must obey natural laws and that it was the task of physiological scientists to find out those laws.

In his early youth, Claude Bernard already proved himself capable of independent thought. He came to Lyon to work as an apothecary's apprentice when he was a young boy, but found little to interest him in mixing salves, making pills and preparing mixtures. He therefore did what all young people do when, like Faust, they feel a world unfolding within themselves; he began to write. No sooner had a little comedy of his been performed in amateur theatricals than he widened his scope further and wrote a tragedy. He tried to find a publisher for it in Paris, but an editor gave him a piece of well-meant advice – that he would do better to go back to his crucibles and pots of salve.

Young Claude, however, had had enough of them. He now decided to study medicine. His rapid rise in this profession proved that he possessed remarkable talent: when his years of study were over he became assistant to the physiologist, François Magendie, at the Hôtel Dieu in Paris. Later, when Magendie advanced to become a professor at the Collège de France, he took young Claude Bernard with him as an amboceptor.

It was Magendie, that master of experimental physiology, who first cleared away the mystical *vitalismus*. In the living organism, only those laws and forces which could be observed in a biological experiment had any validity for him. It was hardly surprising that the master's attitude rubbed off on the pupil; Claude Bernard made experiment after experiment in order to discover the natural laws governing life.

Few people can have any conception what that meant in those days. Modern experimental physiologists have at their disposal palatial laboratories with tiled walls, drains and sinks, with automatic recording apparatus, thermostats and refrigerators, with gleaming instruments and magnificent microscopes...

In comparison, Claude Bernard's so-called laboratory was as a tent is to a luxury villa. It was situated in the cellars of the Collège de France, a damp, dungeon-like hole, and one had to stoop to enter. The research scientist had to make his own equipment; his measuring instruments and recording apparatus; worst of all, experiments on animals, without which physiological research cannot be done, were strictly forbidden by law.

In order to study the problems of digestion and discover the effects of gastric juices, Claude Bernard had inserted a silver tubule into the stomach of a dog and let it heal there, so that he could count on a constant supply of gastric juices. As luck would have it, however, the dog escaped. Bernard was summoned before the commissioner of police and, to his horror, it turned out – misfortunes never come singly – that the dog was the property of the commissioner himself. It had been stolen and then sold to Bernard as a stray. However, sometimes an unfortunate encounter ends well and so it was in this case. The commissioner turned out to be sympathetic to Bernard's predicament. After the circumstances had been explained, the two even became friends and the scientist was able to pursue his work in safety.

In this, and similar ways, pepsin was discovered to be another effective ingredient in gastric juices in addition to hydrochloric acid; the fate of food taken into the organism, its combustion and reconstruction was explored; the secret of the pancreas examined and its chemical composition was compared with that of saliva. Urine, the 'mother substance' of physiological chemistry, was analysed, urea and uric acid were identified, the role played by carbohydrates in metabolism was studied, and 'Bernard's puncture' established that if a certain part of the brain was pricked, it would produce an artificial attack of diabetes. In addition,

Claude Bernard also solved the mystery of the poisonous effect of carbon-monoxide gas which is created if coal is not completely burnt; for, if the red blood corpuscles come into contact with carbon-monoxide, the gas adheres to the red haemochrome with the result that the haemoglobin is rendered incapable of conveying the oxygen vital to life. Claude Bernard was also the first man to introduce the new concept of 'inner secretion' which was to prove so important in years to come. His book, *An Introduction to Experimental Medicine*, which was published in 1865, can be counted as one of the great landmarks in the history of medicine. His country thanked him for his great pioneering achievement by awarding him the greatest honour to which a French scholar can aspire – membership of the Académie Francaise.

The flourishing science of organic chemistry immediately assured the rapid succession of discoveries resulting from this research and, in ever more complicated analyses, tried to find out the chemical construction of all the effective substances in a living organism. The reason why the followers of this new science directed their main endeavours to this particular field may be due to the fact that, among other things, almost all the scientists who assisted at the birth of organic chemistry, came to chemistry from medicine. What was then discovered about the chemistry of metabolism channelled the development of medical science into an entirely new direction; it can even be said to have produced a new outlook on life. The mysterious transformations which the living organism constantly undertakes in its countless tiny chemical laboratories had been moved nearer to comprehension; the mystical 'life force' had been deposed; nevertheless, however many secrets were fathomed, and the more people thought they had discovered, the greater the marvel seemed. Man was forced to recognize ever more clearly that, compared with the chemical foundations of what in its entirety is called life, the most involved and subtle chemical marvels which he can produce in his laboratories and industrial plants are mere child's play.

222

Already it was possible to foresee that one day the range of ideas would come full circle and people become convinced that, in spite of all experiments to explain the organism along scientific lines, the marvel of life could not be explained purely by means of chemico-physical factors.

26

Philippe Pinel of France frees the lunatics and
helps to establish his view that they are not
criminals but sick people. Johann Peter Frank
founds a system of public health welfare.
The English country doctor, Edward
Jenner, develops inoculation with cow-pox
vaccine as a protection against man-pox or
smallpox.

W hen Lazzaro Spallanzani died at the end of the eighteenth century, a new era had begun in the history of the world and of medicine. The stimulating works of Diderot, d'Alembert, La Mettries, Voltaire and Jean-Jacques Rousseau, had ushered in an age of enlightenment and the resultant change in outlook meant that people were no longer comforted by the hope of a better life in the next world; instead, they actively involved themselves in bettering the conditions of life in the present.

In France, the French Revolution was the most visible sign of this struggle which exploded with elemental force; almost as part of it, so to speak, a great medical feat was accomplished which removed a dreadful and abhorrent abuse prevalent at that time: this was the freeing of the insane. This heroic and, in the context of those times, dangerous undertaking, is associated with the name of a French doctor, Philippe Pinel, who was born in 1775, the son of a poor country doctor in Saint-André in the South of France.

People living today can have no conception of the fate confronting mental patients in those days. They were not regarded as sick people but as malevolent criminals or people possessed by the devil and treated accordingly. They were kept like wild animals and, in 1788, Count Mirabeau wrote a pamphlet disclosing the almost incredible conditions which obtained in the Paris lunatic asylum, Bicetre, the one-time prison. 'The new arrivals', he wrote, 'are indiscriminately thrown among this wild crowd of lunatics and from time to time they are shown, like savage beasts, to the first lout who pays his sixpence.' Moreover such conditions were by no means restricted to Paris; in a contemporary travel report from London, for example, it says: 'I and my three little sons went to see the lions, the bridges, the lunatics at Bedlam and other amusing showpieces in the metropolis.'

The treatment of the deranged people was indescribable. They were locked into box-like cages with bars. In order to drive the evil spirits out of them they were whipped with horsewhips or flogged with the birch; they were forced into straitjackets or covered cribs in which they could not move, or they were punished by being made to stand for hours chained to the wall with their arms outstretched, the upper part of their body pulled up on a rope so that only their toes still touched the ground. The most dreadful torture, however, was the 'turning chair'. The mental patients were tied to it and then, by means of special machinery, made to turn at a great speed. Ice-cold showerbaths and plunge-baths up to three hundred times a day complemented the inhuman treatment; gags and face-masks prevented people from hearing the shrieks and cries of the victims.

Pinel, who had come to medicine from philosophy and theology, was appointed director of the Bicetre Asylum in Paris in 1792. A personal experience caused him to undertake its reform. A close friend suddenly developed a psychosis and was sent to Bicetre. His terror of the treatment meted out was so great that he fled into the forests near Paris where he fell victim to the wolves.

His friend's tragic fate stirred Pinel's conscience. He told himself that if a man went to his death rather than to Bicetre then the treatment must be as inhuman as the estimate of the mental patient. At a time when the equality of men was solemnly being proclaimed on the Champs de Mars, Pinel, unafraid, came before the Assembly and demanded the same rights for his deranged inmates.

At first, as can be imagined, he encountered considerable scepticism, especially as the people exercising the revolutionary power feared that among those locked up in Bicetre there might well turn out to be enemies of the Republic. Nevertheless, Pinel succeeded in persuading the head of the Commune, a man called Gouthon, to visit the asylum. When Gouthon saw the horde of chained-up, howling and raving patients, he was so taken aback he told Pinel: 'You must be mad yourself, Citizen Pinel, if you demand that these beasts should be unchained.'

However Pinel was not to be discouraged. He would not give up and continued to put forward his request with kindly obstinacy. Thanks to his reputation in other branches of the arts, he succeeded in establishing his view that madness was not a crime but a disease; and he supported this conception by publishing a medico-philosophical book about mental illness. After that, the fate of the wretched mental cases was radically changed. The excellent French School of Psychiatry developed Pinel's ideas still further; the prisons for psychotics turned into hospitals in which humane methods of treatment were employed.

If the freeing of the mental cases was in some measure already part of the public health system which can also be set to the credit of the era of enlightenment, further medical exploits took place around the same time, the benefits of which were not felt just by individuals so much as by the whole population. It was left to a doctor from the Rhineland, Johann Peter Frank, to create a comprehensive state health welfare system. 'The inner security of the State', said Frank, 'is the object of the public police intelligence; a very considerable part of this is to know how to manage the health welfare of people living in communities, and that of the animals which they need for their work and subsistence, according to certain laws...'

These words heralded nothing less than a new era in medical history and particularly in that branch of medicine which is concerned with public hygiene, health welfare, with what we would today call sanitary inspectors and with official measures to prevent disease, epidemics, plagues, etc.

Johann Peter Frank was one of those figures in medical history whose ideas were far ahead of their times. He clearly recognized that, with all deference to the sciences, they did not end with anatomy, physiology and pathology, but that prevention was at least as important as the recognition and treatment of disease.

He seemed almost predestined to fulfil the task of moulding these ideas into a system and, to this end, arranging the necessary measures into a magnificent comprehensive sanitation plan; for, with a brilliant talent for observation, he combined love of humanity and scientific perspicacity.

Doubtless, in addition to all this, the experience of his own childhood played a part in making him especially suited to the task he had set himself.

He was born on 19 March 1745 in Rodalben in the Rhenish Palatinate, the son of the manager of a glass works and, as he had no less than thirteen brothers and sisters, he soon gained personal experience of the difficulties of life. It was not at all easy for his father to let him study, but as Johann Peter was an intelligent boy, the impossible was made possible and, in order to prepare for a clerical career, he studied philosophy in Metz and Pont-à-Mousson and took his degree in that subject.

However, the young graduate felt an irresistible urge to occupy himself with the natural sciences and medicine so, to the dismay of his parents, he started a second course of study at Heidelberg and Strasbourg and eventually graduated as a doctor of medicine as well.

At that time, an idea was already taking root in his mind for the creation of an interrelated scientific system out of those official measures which helped to promote general health care, the fight against infectious diseases and the prevention of plagues and epidemics. But the poor young doctor first had to earn his own living before he could think of realizing such ambitious plans. He practised medicine in Bitsch and Rastatt, became district physician of Baden-Baden, town and country physician in Bruchsal and, meanwhile, returned to his self-imposed task whenever the opportunity arose.

He gave it the wide-ranging title: *A Systematic and Comprehensive Medical Policy* and, in 1779 – when the author was thirty-four years old – the first volume of this monumental handbook was published. It dealt with the problems of reproduction, touched on the healthy influence the 'delights of dancing' had upon young girls, spoke out against the celibacy of the Catholic clergy and was far ahead of the times in uttering a warning that people with severe inherited weaknesses should seek the advice of a doctor before marrying.

The problem of illegitimate children, venereal diseases, etc., was covered in the second volume which appeared in 1780; and the third volume, which came out three years later, concentrated on nutrition, dress and domestic hygiene.

Meanwhile, interest was aroused in scientific circles as Johann Peter's books enjoyed a wide distribution. A year after the third volume had appeared, he was appointed professor of philosophy and medical policy first in Göttingen and, another year later, in Pavia, where he could then put his revolutionary ideas into practice and reform the entire medical system of Lombardy.

In the meantime, the fourth volume devoted to forensic medicine appeared in 1788.

In 1795, the restless man became director of the General Hospital in Vienna; in 1804 he lectured at the University of Vilna and, a year later, he was appointed personal physician to Tsar Alexander in St Petersburg.

However, he only stayed there for three years; then he turned up in Vienna again where, for the time being, he ended his work in 1814 with volume five which discussed questions involving medical jurisprudence and, finally, dealt with the burial of corpses.

Johann Peter Frank now spent the rest of his stormy, restless life in Vienna. He finished his work once and for all and crowned it with a sixth volume which dealt with 'the art of healing in general and of the influence thereof on the welfare of the state'. He died on 24 April 1821, justly described as 'one of the most important doctors of all time' and, above all, as 'the founder of public health welfare'.

At this point in medical history the idea that greater emphasis should be placed upon the prevention of diseases rather than on their diagnosis and treatment could no longer be ignored; it reached its classical culmination in the person of the English doctor, Edward Jenner. It is thanks to his work that the terror of smallpox was removed, the dreadful scourge of mankind, which had been so terrifyingly widespread in Europe and accounted for about a tenth of the total mortality of the Continent; it is thanks to him, too, that an outbreak of smallpox which, not more than a century earlier, would have killed about half a million people in a Europe still sparsely populated in comparison with today, now only consists of a few sporadic, isolated cases which are generally imported as a result of air-traffic with the East.

Jenner was born on 17 May 1749, the son of a clergyman in Berkeley, Gloucestershire. First he served his apprenticeship with a surgeon in Sudbury near Bristol. Then, when he was twenty-one, he entered London University and, after completing his studies, settled down as a doctor in Berkeley.

His professional duties frequently took him to the estates which were situated near his country home; there he had to inoculate the men and maidservants against smallpox which was generally done by letting pus of variola dry on the end of threads and then introducing the 'weakened' smallpox virus into scratches made in the skin. For experience had shown that as a result of a 'variolation' of this kind, people went through a milder, local form of this disease and remained protected for the rest of their lives against the serious, mortal and disfiguring general disease.

During his variolations, Jenner noticed time and again that in some people the inoculation disease took a more or less acute course, while others suffered no inoculation disease at all, and, as he was an intelligent man with acute powers of observation, who was used to probing a question to the limit, he was soon on the right track. This pointed towards cows who frequently suffered from a pustular illness affecting the udders which was very like human smallpox in appearance. It was therefore called cow-pox (*Variolae vaccinae*) and could also be transmitted to humans who, however, suffered no injury as a result, except for a few harmless local pustules.

Again and again it was confirmed that those menservants and maids on whom the smallpox inoculations had no effect had previously suffered an attack of cow-pox, sometimes a great many years earlier. Jenner found out that country folk were well aware of this relationship when he wanted to 'variolate' a young maid and she told him there was no need as she had already had cow-pox and so could never get smallpox.

At that moment Jenner had the great flash of inspiration which today strikes us as so obvious, but which nevertheless represents such a monumental step forward: why inoculate people with the dangerous smallpox virus which, in spite of every care, could be quite unpredictable? Why not use the harmless cow-pox virus instead?

However, Edward Jenner was much too careful and responsible a man to publish his discovery right away. He spent several more years checking his discovery, observing and making numerous experiments; but when at last he informed the Royal Society of Sciences in London of what he had found, the result was just as could be expected: those worthy men sitting round the green table turned up their noses and laughed at the unknown country doctor.

He did not let this annoy him, however, particularly as other people had, by now, also become aware of the fact that an attack of cow-pox could safeguard a man from smallpox. Thus it is not unimportant to know that in 1791, a teacher in Holstein, Plett by name, was already successfully protecting children against smallpox by inoculating them with cow-pox.

However, even when, seven years later, in 1798, Edward Jenner published his observations in a book, the time was still not ripe and another number of years had to pass before they received general recognition.

Then, at last, Jenner's idea triumphed. In 1802 parliament presented the indefatigable champion of vaccination with an honorarium amounting to ten thousand pounds which, a few years later, was followed by another of thirty thousand pounds; and now protective vaccination with cow-pox became the public property of all civilized nations. The dangerous inoculation or 'variolation' with the virus of the real smallpox became the innocuous 'vaccination' which – despite all criticisms – has brought an immeasurable blessing to mankind.

Edward Jenner died in Berkeley, his home town, on 26 January 1823, highly respected and honoured as a benefactor to mankind. In 1857 the grateful British people put up a monument to him, now to be found in Kensington Gardens in London; the marble statue by Monteverde representing Jenner vaccinating a child, is particularly famous.

27

*The Frenchman, Xavier Bichat, establishes
general anatomy through his 'theory of
membranes'. Corvisart, Napoleon's personal
physician, amplifies Auenbrugger's physical
method of diagnostics. Laennec invents the
stethoscope.*

While the great revolution still
raged in France, the obsolete medical faculty in Paris, which had
long ago been overtaken by those in Leiden, Vienna and
Göttingen, had been swept away by events. However, the French
Revolution did not merely destroy; it also constructed. Under
the direction of a far-sighted doctor and chemist, Antoine François
de Fourcroy, who was a member both of the National Assembly
and the Committee of Public Safety, and who carried through a
regulation governing uniformity of weights and measures, three
schools of medicine were created in Paris, Montpellier and
Strasbourg, to which special hospitals for the instruction of
students were attached. In one stroke France had replaced her
Paris faculty, which was still living in the past, with the most up-
to-date establishments for medical instruction and research; and,
as a result of this reorganization, French medicine took an undisputed lead in medical progress for a long time to come.

Pierre-Joseph Desault, who was the head surgeon of the Hôtel
Dieu and one of the most outstanding surgeons of his time, was
appointed director of the new Ecole de Santé. He had been

arrested in 1793 in the middle of a lecture, but had been set free again after only a few days. Desault can be said to have founded the science of topographical anatomy; but practical surgery also owes many improvements to him. To this day, Desault's bandage for the clavicle bears the name of its originator. Moreover Desault's school became an eloquent proof of the fresh wind which had been blowing through the medical faculty following the Revolution, and also since the National Assembly had demanded of the professors that they should further the progress of medical science by their own research.

This summons was nowhere more effective than with a young, ambitious medical student who was one of Desault's favourite pupils: Marie François Xavier Bichat. He, too, was a child of the French Revolution and, after he had made a brief meteoric career, fate was to lay him low. However the lifespan allotted to him was sufficient for him to achieve a place of honour in the history book of medicine.

Bichat was born in 1771, the son of a country doctor in a Jura village; and since he already showed an early interest in anatomy and physiology, there was never any doubt that he, too, would follow the medical profession. He began his medical studies in Montpellier and Lyons; but just after he had mastered the rudiments of anatomy and physiology, he was, in common with almost all his fellow students, caught up in the Revolution and conscripted into the army. Then, in 1793 – the same year in which Louis XVI's head was struck off by the guillotine in the Place de la Concorde – destiny took him to Paris where the genius of this twenty-two-year-old student was to be fulfilled in a short, meteoric flight, before being extinguished for ever when he was not yet thirty.

Just as a seemingly insignificant event often lifts one of life's favourites out of the crowd so, too, it happened here. In the Desault clinic it was the custom for an advanced student to recapitulate in a lecture the subjects which had most recently been studied. When, on one such occasion, the chosen candidate was missing, a young student – Xavier Bichat – announced that he was ready to give the lecture in his place. The head of the clinic gave his assent; the students and probationers smiled for they anticipated a glorious fiasco. But Bichat had only been speaking, without notes, for a short while, when their laughter changed to amazement. They sensed that here was a great talent awaiting development and at once Bichat – although normally a shy person – had everyone on his side. Above all, Desault, who had at once recognized his outstanding gifts, gave him active assistance.

A brilliant career would have lain before Xavier Bichat if the saying – that those whom the gods favour they take early into their keeping – had not applied to him, too. He founded the Medical Society for scientific competition and at the turn of the century could be found at the famous Hôtel Dieu of Paris. From then on he could pursue his real preference – the study of anatomy and physiology – to his heart's content. However, it seemed as if the intensely burning flame was consuming this highly gifted young man. He never left the autopsy theatre or laboratory and, like Vesalius, dissected, laid out, experimented and wrote without pause day and night ...

During one winter he dissected no less than six hundred corpses; then however, his exhausted body, which he drove so relentlessly, avenged itself. He began to sicken, consumption stretched out its claws for him. Yet a feverish urgency in him, as in all sufferers of tuberculosis, who sense they have no time to lose, drove him on to ever greater efforts. Then, at last, came the breakdown. At thirty, he had to lay aside scalpel and pen for ever.

It is astonishing how much Xavier Bichat managed to accomplish during his short active life; he left behind four great medical works. One dealt with general, another with specific anatomy. Yet another with physiological inquiries into life and death. His greatest, most pioneering work, however, was his treatise on the tissues. For it was Xavier Bichat who, for the first time, systematically and methodically examined the human body from the point of view of the different substances out of which it is built. He recognized that there were a number of different tissues – he called them membranes – and by tracing them back to a series of basic forms, made the further discovery that such tissues could be found in all the different organs or parts of the body; moreover that the specific texture of such membranes constantly recurs in the fine structure of the sections of the body. He thus became the founder of a branch of science known as general anatomy. This achievement was all the more remarkable as at that time the animal cell had not yet been discovered.

Xavier Bichat's theory of membranes recognized a comparatively large number of different tissues in the human body; he distinguished between no less than twenty-one basic membranes. From his experience, he concluded that not only was normal vitality located in the membranes but also the vitality of disease and, supporting his anatomical idea with this assumption, he established it in pathology. Typical of this attitude was Bichat's dictum: 'Several post-mortems shed more light than twenty years' observation of symptoms'. Moreover he was anything but a bleak materialist. He remained steadfast in the opinion that physiological processes are different from physical ones and that life is subject to its own laws.

Yet another great doctor emerged from the Desault school in those restless times: Jean Nicolas Corvisart, born in 1755. As the son of a public prosecutor he was actually intended for the law, but the study of jurisprudence bored him so much that he began to frequent medical lectures. When he heard Desault speak in the Hôtel Dieu, he was completely carried away. The experience proved decisive. Corvisart turned from the study of law to that of medicine.

He underwent his training in Desault's hospital, ending in 1782; and then began his medical career miserably as a 'poor doctor' for practically nothing; it was not until he joined the staff of the Neckar Hospital that things improved. In contrast to his master, Desault, he concentrated more and more on internal medicine, accepted a position in the Charité, and, after a few years, became its director.

Corvisart was especially interested in the 'percussion' method (see page 211) which had been invented about forty years earlier by Leopold Auenbrugger. He translated and extended Auenbrugger's work *Inventum Novum*; he perfected the technique of percussion and furthered medical research by describing in the minutest detail how the different varieties of heart disease could be distinguished by this method.

Meanwhile the Revolution had been superseded by the Napoleonic regime; Corvisart, the erstwhile poor doctor, who was by now also professor of practical medicine at the Collège de France, became the great Corsican's personal physician. The time for research and study was over; the social obligations of the new imperial court reached such proportions that there was even hardly any time left for medicine. Corvisart resigned; nevertheless his name is remembered in the history of medicine. That he was a great doctor not just in the medical sense but also from the human point of view is best shown by the words of that great sceptic, Napoleon, who once said: 'I don't believe in medicine. I believe in Corvisart'.

In any event, Corvisart's name would be memorable if only for having a pupil who gave practical medicine the second most used instrument after the clinical thermometer – the stethoscope. His name was René Théophile Hyacinthe Laennec. This industrious and imaginative promoter of medical science is worth mention if alone for the fact that while still only young he courageously sacrificed his own life in the furtherance of medical knowledge.

Laennec was born on 17 February 1781 at Quimper in Brittany. He grew up during the troubled years of the French Revolution. He spent his childhood with an uncle in Nantes and there he may have acquired the germ of his preference for a medical career. When the revolutionary disorders spread through the land, his uncle was called up to serve in the field hospital of the western army and young René, who had already acquired his first schooling in Nantes, accompanied his foster father in the capacity of what we would now call medical orderly. Thus, he got to know the medical profession from the bottom up and, when he entered the University of Paris in 1800 in order to study medicine, he was already familiar with most of the elementary concepts of medical science as it then was.

Laennec soon left his fellow students behind; he eclipsed them with his attainments and won his doctor's degree after barely four years' study. He received an appointment at the Beaujon Hospital scarcely eight years after he became a doctor and, shortly afterwards, he was also appointed to the Salpêtrière. He had just reached his thirty-fifth year when he became medical superintendent of the Neckar Hospital, and now he had everything he needed in order to pursue research to his heart's content. True, in doing so he demanded too much of his never too strong constitution; and his creative spirit was sometimes so indefatigable that it almost seemed as if he knew that there was not much more time at his disposal.

Laennec's discovery of the stethoscope which made his name famous in medical history was arrived at in a strange way. One day when he was strolling through the courtyard of the Louvre, he watched some children clambering about on a pile of beams. He saw two of them communicate with each other at a distance: one child holding its ear against one end of a beam and the second one knocking out signals at the other end.

At once Laennec had a flash of inspiration. It must be possible, he said to himself, to make the tone of the organs in the chest, the beating of the heart and the sound of breathing in the lungs, more audible by using a similar method. Quite apart from the possibility of a more subtle diagnosis, such a procedure would also be of positive benefit to an examining doctor, for there were patients in the Neckar Hospital on whose chest no doctor would enjoy laying his ear. In his zeal for work Laennec had done so year in year out without the slightest consideration for his own health; he was to pay for his unselfish research work with his life!

No sooner had the young doctor returned to the hospital than he set about putting his idea into practice. He was in such a hurry that he did not wait for a wooden instrument to be made, but took a few sheets of writing paper, rolled them into a tube, set one end of it on the chest of the patient and placed his ear on the other end. What he had hoped for happened. He could now hear the tones of the heart and the sound of breathing in the lungs appreciably more clearly.

From the makeshift paper roll to the wooden tube was but a step; the stethoscope without which a modern doctor can hardly be imagined had been discovered, auscultation of the organs in the chest had moved an immense step forward, diagnosis of all lung and heart diseases had been decisively improved. However, Laennec was much too conscientious a researcher to be satisfied with what he had achieved. He was anxious to verify wherever possible what he had found and so he made post-mortem examinations on all patients who had died of diseases affecting the organs in the chest, to see whether what he had established by means of his new stethoscope while they were alive was proved correct in the corpse.

Three years passed in indefatigable, one might almost say hectic, work of this kind; the fruit of this unflinching labour on the living and the dead, the two extensive volumes of the work *Traité de l'auscultation médiate et des maladies des poumons et du coeur*, appeared in 1819. However, when Laennec had got the results of his devoted research written down, he was at the end of his powers of resistance. He collapsed and had to give up his medical work for a time and went to his beloved Brittany to recuperate. There, he enjoyed the retirement of an Arcadian country life, took pleasure in reading the ancient writers and tried to penetrate into the secrets of the Celtic language.

This idyll lasted two years; then there was no keeping the barely convalescent man in his native province. In 1822 he was back in Paris again. Meanwhile, his system had gained ground; he was granted the professorship in practical medicine at the Collège de France and, a year later, made professor of clinical medicine at the University of Paris. Laennec's name became ever more widely known; doctors came to the French capital from all over the world in order to learn the new practice of auscultation from the man who had himself invented it. But destiny only granted Laennec a few more years. When he had finished the second, still more voluminous edition of his work in 1826, he again fell ill. Once again he tried to find convalescence and recovery in his Breton home country; but the germ of consumption with which he had become infected during his untiring examinations at the sick-bed had, in the meantime, gained ground. On 13 August 1826, Laennec died in Kerlouanec near Douameney in Brittany at the age of forty-five, the unselfish victim of his research. His invention of the stethoscope, which has since become a positive symbol of the doctor, was complementary to a degree to the physical methods of medical diagnosis developed by Leopold Auenbrugger with his system of percussion and continued so logically by Jean Nicolas Corvisart.

A description of the French clinicians who made medical history before, during and after the French Revolution would not be complete without mentioning a pupil of Pinel, Bichat and Corvisart who, for a time, enjoyed great medical authority in spite of the fact that, with scarcely believable prejudice, he led medical science into a hopeless cul-de-sac. His name was François Joseph Victor Broussais. He was, in character, the opposite of the sensitive, musical Laennec; a robust, gruff man who was also a Breton.

In 1792, at the age of twenty, he became a soldier, a true son of the Revolution, a rabid atheist; as fiery an adherent of Napoleon as he was a bitter enemy of the royal house. He accompanied the emperor on his campaigns through thick and thin; then, after completing his studies, he became a military doctor and later, the head of a military hospital in Paris.

While pathologists were concentrating more and more on breaking down the concept of disease by drawing up clear, distinct, clinical pictures and finding in the body the seat of various diseases, Broussais roughly tore down the whole carefully constructed edifice. He announced that there were no such things as different individual diseases; for him every disease depended basically on the same process which sometimes occurred in a milder and sometimes in a more severe form and manifested itself now in this part of the body and now in that. All diseases could be traced back to inflammations and these practically always had their origin in the gastro-intestinal canal. The only sensible therapy, therefore, was to attack the inflammation in this organic system; and this was done with leeches.

Broussais, who had at his disposal great powers of persuasion, won many adherents for his peculiar system. As a result, the demand for leeches became prodigious: in 1827 thirty-three million leeches were imported into France; in 1833 the number was forty-three million. Fortunately, an opponent to Broussais was soon to appear in the person of Pierre Charles Alexandre Louis, born in 1787, who introduced the science of statistics into medicine. By means of these he easily proved that Broussais' universal remedies of bleeding and applying leeches were not only useless for many diseases, but often even harmful.

In spite of the errors of Broussaism, the Parisian medical school, which had, as a result of its achievements, acquired world-wide prestige, continued to play a leading role in clinical medicine for quite a long time to come. Meanwhile, the coming age, when doctors would recognize that many diseases were caused by minute organisms and were therefore infectious, began to cast a growing shadow. Pierre Bretonneau of Tours was the first to recognize the infectious nature of diphtheria and enteric fever; however, this was disputed by most of his colleagues.

Other famous clinicians belonging to the then Paris school are remembered by medical terms now in daily use. Thus, the artificial liberation of spasms in tetany by pressure on the nerve trunks is called Trousseau's phenomenon after the Paris clinician, Armand Trousseau, who lived from 1801 to 1867; and the most important French surgeon of that time was Guillaume Dupuytren (1777–1835) after whom was named the inflammatory, cicatrically contracted aponeurosis of the palm. Finally, Hodgkin's disease or lymphogranulomatosis takes its name from Laennec's pupil, Thomas Hodgkin (1798–1864), who helped to ensure that the progress achieved by the French medical school was also transmitted to England.

The new clinical medicine did not gain acceptance in the German-speaking countries until shortly before the middle of the nineteenth century, when the Viennese medical school which, since Gerard van Swieten and Anton de Haen (see page 207), had gradually sunk into another enchanted hundred years' sleep, experienced a revival due to certain outstanding doctors. But more will be said of this in Chapter 30.

28

Matthias Jakob Schleiden discovers the
plant cells; Johannes Evangelista Purkinje
recognizes them as 'elementary constituents'.
Theodor Schwann extends the new
histology of cells to cover the whole realm
of living creatures and human beings. The
focus on the cell nucleus leads on from a
predominantly statical method of observa-
tion to a distinctly dynamic mode of
thought.

Following Xavier Bichat's theory
of membranes, which was discussed at the beginning of the previous chapter, anatomical research also began to try to penetrate
still further into the secrets of the structural elements of the
human body. Already during the seventeenth century, while
examining various objects from the plant or animal world through
his home-made microscope, Antonius van Leeuwenhoek (see
Chapter 20) had occasionally come across various structures which
did not seem to consist of uniform compact material, but of a
larger or smaller number of similarly formed elements. He called
these organic elements 'little dumplings' and just as superficialities
can sometimes influence the pursuit of an idea, so it may have
been due to Leeuwenhoek's scarcely well-chosen description that
no one attributed much significance to his observation.

Marcello Malpighi had apparently also seen the strange elementary particles. However, being an ardent phytotomist, the versatile Italian founder of microscopic anatomy observed them chiefly in plants. About the same time as Malpighi was applying himself to his studies in Bologna, in Northern Europe an English physicist, Robert Hooke, was busy examining various natural objects of animal and vegetable origin under the microscope, as was rapidly becoming fashionable. Besides mosses and lichens, insects and spiders, he also chose to examine a piece of elderberry pith. He cut it into fine, transparent little slices and when he examined one of these paper-thin discs under the microscope, he saw that the tissue consisted of numerous little alveolar chambers ranged side by side. The same phenomenon repeated itself when he examined thin slices of cork; here, too, he found that the material was composed of numerous little identical parts. He called them 'cells' without realizing how important this description would become in the future; for the whole modern theory of life would be inconceivable without this idea of the cell. It was not until the middle of the last century that two German research scientists built what had so far been regarded as a chance observation into a closely knit system: cytology. One of the two scientists was called Matthias Jakob Schleiden; he helped one of the most significant pieces of the previous century's biological reasoning to triumph. Born in Hamburg in 1804, he first studied jurisprudence, but instinct soon told him that law was not his subject. Therefore he changed over to botany although he had already gained a doctorate in law. His methodical studies soon convinced him that all plant organisms were composed of numerous tiny and basically similar elements, or cells. He was also especially interested in the formation of the cells and soon found out that the nucleus inside the cell played a decisive role. In 1838 when he was thirty-four, he published an essay on *Phytogenesis*, or the origin of plants.

A year earlier, in 1837, the Czech, Johannes Evangelista Purkinje – one of the most versatile research scientists of modern times, appointed on Goethe's recommendation to be professor of physiology and pathology in Breslau in 1823 – had identified the cells as being the primary components of a plant; therefore Purkinje should justly count as the co-founder of histology.

Since it seemed rather far-fetched and insufficiently established to the official botanists, Schleiden's essay would probably have sunk into obscurity without trace if it had not – by what might appear to be a lucky chance, but actually because the time was ripe for it – fallen into the hands of an extremely open-minded young anatomist from Berlin called Theodor Schwann.

Schwann was born in 1810 at Neuss on the Rhine, the fourth son of a bookseller and publisher. The family was a large one: Theodor had no less than twelve brothers and sisters. Although Schwann's adolescence coincided with an era of colossal progress in the natural sciences, especially in physics and chemistry, he stayed a devout Catholic and in order not to anger his church, obtained the permission of the Archbishop of Mecheln before publishing his writings.

He buried himself in his work in a dark backroom in the centre of Berlin, far from all social activities; he studied, prepared specimens, examined through his microscope and experimented. In 1834 he also took his state medical examination and then became the assistant, at the Anatomical Institute, of the famous physician, anatomist, physiologist, and pathologist, Johannes Müller, of whom a more detailed account will be given later (see Chapter 32). Not much could be done on a salary of ten thalers a month, but young Schwann did not have expensive tastes. In his spare time he preferred to work in his hermit's cell; sometimes he did not leave his room for days.

Fate decreed that Schleiden's *Phytogenesis* should fall into Schwann's hands; and on the thoughtful young man – who also got to know Schleiden personally – the reading of this work on the history of plants acted like a catalyst calling forth a turbulent chemical reaction. Suddenly, it was as if scales had fallen from his eyes: he was sure he had detected the same basic elements Schleiden was describing for all plant organisms during his own microscopic examination of animal and human tissue. Now it was only one step to the realization that animal and human organisms were also composed of countless such tiny basic elements; indeed, were not in general many of the basic elements such as are to be found in animal and human body fluids – for example the blood corpuscles, the spermatozoa and others – really unicellular organisms?

In 1839, less than a year after the publication of Schleiden's work, Theodor Schwann brought out his book *Microscopic Examinations of the Conformity in Structure and Growth of Plants and Animals*. This time the work, in which the twenty-nine-year-old man extended the histology of plant cells to include the whole world of living organisms, did not fail to produce an impact. Its publication became a turning-point in the entire field of organic sciences; anatomy and physiology – with it, research on the human being – were placed on an entirely new basis. The simplest organisms, which had already been observed by Leeuwenhoek – and which we now know only consisted of one cell – had, so to speak, stayed at the lowest stage of development. All higher forms of life, however, were formed of a 'cell-state'. The human organism is one such gigantic 'cell-state' in which each individual cell has its own special function; the cell-state can only exist as a result of the harmonious cooperation of all its elements. That which we call life, however, is bound up with the metabolism of the cell; consequently the cell is the ultimate bearer of life...

Thus Purkinje, Schleiden and Schwann's histology of cells led on from the hitherto predominantly statical way of thinking to a distinctly dynamic one by drawing attention to the cell nucleus and recognizing its significance with regard to the continuous creation of new cells. Schwann's definition, according to which all plant and animal cells possess a cellular membrane, was questioned for a long time. Only the existence of a cellular membrane for plants was allowed, animal cells being denied the existence of a membrane of their own. Schwann's assumption could only quite recently be confirmed in its entirety when the electron microscope revealed that there is no such thing as a cell without a cellular membrane.

Schwann's book won wide renown, and histology of cells had a more lasting influence on biology than any other previous discovery. The fact that it was also to become the starting-point for a pathology of its own – cellular pathology – will be remembered when Rudolf Virchow's life and works are described (see page 279).

29

*Luigi Galvani discovers 'animal electricity'
and believes that by doing so he has solved
the riddle of life. The 'outsider' of
medicine: Franz Anton Mesmer and his
magnetism. Joseph Gall and phrenology;
Samuel Hahnemann and homeopathy; the
disruption of medical development at the
turn of the nineteenth century.*

There is no discipline among the
arts in which the so-called 'outsider' thrives so well as in medicine.
For as long as scientific medicine has been taught in universities,
attempts have been made to damn it, to dispose of it as 'unnatural'
and to replace it by one speculative system or another. It was
as certain as night follows day that the immense progress achieved,
particularly in the second half of the eighteenth century, in all
fields of natural science – in physics and chemistry, in anatomy,
physiology, histology, etc., would call forth a reaction against
the all too rational and materialistic attitudes in medical affairs.
It is by no means a unique event in medical history that attitudes
went to the opposite extreme.

The stimulus for this kind of development was given – quite
unconsciously – by a professor of anatomy and practical doctor
in Bologna called Luigi Galvani. As the result of a chance observation, he arrived at one of the most momentous and impor-

tant scientific achievements produced during the eighteenth century.

Galvani was born on 9 September 1737 in Bologna and it was there, too, that at the end of his schooldays he began the study of medicine and the natural sciences. He remained faithful to his home town; when he was not yet twenty-five he gave lectures and a few years later was a professor at the famous Northern Italian university.

It was his hobby to study the physiology of the nerves which control the muscular system; and since frogs were in good supply as animals suitable for research, he made experiments using the skinned legs of freshly killed batrachians as specimens. While carrying out this work in 1780 he made a startling observation. Near the table on which he was doing his experiments stood a static electricity machine, and whenever a spark was induced in it, the frogs' leg specimens gave a violent jerk if the metal scalpel used came into contact with a femoral nerve.

Galvani, the born research scientist, sensed with intuitive genius that here was something new, that he had witnessed the first signs of something extremely important and at once he was gripped by the excitement of discovery. 'The matter began in this way,' he wrote. 'I was dissecting a frog, had prepared it and laid it out, ignoring everything else, on a table on which there was also an electricity machine. When one of the people assisting me happened by chance to touch the inner femoral nerves quite lightly with the point of a scalpel, all the muscles at the joints appeared to shrink together as if they had been seized by a violent cramp. This fired me with an unbelievable eagerness and desire to put the remarkable phenomenon more closely to the test and to bring to light what it concealed.'

What he had observed so gripped Galvani that he continued making stimulus experiments on the frogs' leg specimens for more than ten years. Again, it was a chance observation which led him in the right direction. One day, while he was working out-of-doors, he hung the prepared frogs' legs from their nerve-ends by iron hooks on the railings of his balcony. A puff of wind blew them against the iron railing and, every time they touched, although there was no electric machine nearby, they gave a violent jerk.

At once Galvani sensed that a lucky chance had shown him an entirely new source of electricity. 'I have', he reported, 'made many experiments on the frogs' legs with different metals, in other rooms, and at various different times of day, and always with the same result. The jerks could only be differentiated among the different metals by the fact that some were weaker and others stronger.' In spite of his inherent modesty, and in his excitement over his discovery, Galvani believed that the last remaining riddle of life had been solved by the electrical phenomena. He thought that the brains of humans and animals produced an electric 'fluid' and that this reached the muscles via the blood-vessels and 'nerve tubes' which were then thought to exist.

Although Galvani's ideas may have seemed somewhat fantastic, they were not fantastic enough for his contemporary, Franz Anton Mesmer, born in 1714 at Iznang on Lake Constance. Mesmer, who began as a theologian and then turned to medicine, took his doctor's degree in Vienna in 1755 with a thesis *De Influxu Planetarum in Corpus Humanum* (About the influence of the planets on the human body). In Vienna, Mesmer started a profitable practice. He introduced the magnet as an item of medical equipment – which, by the way, Paracelsus had already done two-and-a-half centuries earlier – and taught that a 'magnetic fluid' existed inside humans. The power of magnetism was, it is true, restricted to certain special doctors among whom he, Mesmer, was naturally included. By means of stroking, touching and laying on of hands – reminiscent of the ancient method of healing scrofula practised by French and English kings – the magnetizing doctor was able to cause the magnetic force to become active and so heal his patient. It was even supposed to be enough for the magnetist to concentrate his will on the healing of his patient for the healing power of the magnetic fluid to become active in the sufferer.

Healers who know how to convince people of something new, be it never so strange, have always been able to attract crowds; so the magnetic practice of the miracle doctor Mesmer flourished in an unprecedented way. Nevertheless, in spite of the suggestive force of his personality, which is, after all, the basis of all psychotherapeutic success, he did run into trouble. He made it known that his magnetic methods had enabled a blind girl to see and, when this turned out to be a downright swindle, he had to leave Vienna overnight.

Mesmer rapidly transferred the scene of his operations to Paris and it was not long before he was considered just as fashionable there as he had been in the imperial city on the Danube. It also became clear that magnetism was anything but an unprofitable occupation. Mesmer acquired highly respected patients and his practice became more affluent than ever. He achieved his biggest coup, however, when he promised to reveal his healing method to all contributors paying a subscription. This 'subscription' brought him no less than 340,000 livres!

However, he never made the promised revelation. Since several people in high positions died after his treatment – probably not so much because of his healing methods but because of the time wasted before applying an effective therapy – the authorities concerned themselves with Mesmerism. Two commissions were set up and both pronounced the opinion that Mesmer's so-called magnetism 'was void of all reality and the work of an overexcited imagination even if it was not intentional fraud'. There for the time being, the fashionable cure of Mesmerism seemed to end; its founder was banished from France, returned to Germany and died in Meersburg on Lake Constance in 1815.

In Germany, Mesmerism chiefly became popular through the work of the writer, Johann Kaspar Lavater, who was born in Zurich in 1741. Mesmerism fitted well into Lavater's passionate mysticism. He had been Goethe's friend for a time and engaged in a correspondence with him. Meanwhile, it was Lavater's ambition to make a personal contribution to science. He believed he could obtain reliable evidence of a man's character and mental attitude by studying the outline of his profile and, in learned words, advertised his attempt to acquire for physiognomy the status of a true science. In fact his many-volumed work *Physiognomical Fragments* for a short time made him quite famous. However, it is true to say that Goethe soon recognized the weaknesses in Lavater's theory of physiognomy. In a conversation with Eckermann he said: 'Lavater was a sincerely good man, but he was subject to great delusions and the whole stern truth was not his affair; he lied to himself and to others.'

Evidently the idea of finding details of a man's character from his outward appearance was popular at that time. This attempt resulted in an entirely new fashionable science, created by a man whose ideas were not based on mystical or magical speculations, but on the firm ground of scientific anatomy. His name was Franz Joseph Gall; he was born in 1758 in Tiefbronn near Pforzheim. Gall was already interested in the relationship between special talents and the shape of the skull when he was only a student. After he had graduated as a doctor of medicine in Vienna in 1785 and acquired a flourishing practice there, his hobby was still the study of the brain and shape of the skull.

The longer Gall observed, the more convinced he became that the different functions of the mind were located in different sections of the cerebral cortex and that the greater or lesser development of one part of the brain or another must be reflected in the mental activity which belonged to it. From this conviction, it was but a step to the assumption that the greater development of a particular section of the brain must be noticeable on its outer side, since the formation of the skull must fit itself to the surface of the brain. In other words, it should be possible to tell the mental qualities of a man from the outer shape of his skull, and to deduce his capabilities, impulses, tendencies, character traits, etc.

As can be imagined, Gall's theory – called 'phrenology' in England – caused a great sensation, since it went so far to meet everyone's desires. Soon, particularly because of the over-zealous efforts of many of Gall's followers, 'phrenology' became as fashionable a 'science' as Mesmer's magnetism. Whether the story that King Frederick William of Prussia invited Gall to Potzdam and presented him with a number of disguised criminals for skull diagnosis is true or not is doubtful. It is a fact that he was commanded to come to Potzdam and give a lecture there. He himself wrote about it on 3 May 1805: 'In Potzdam all the officers in the Prussian Army, together with the brothers of the King and Queen, are to hear me. That is a splendid martial audience of more than two hundred soldiers.'

It would take too long to mention all the other men who, during the eighteenth century, brought into being comparatively short-lived doctrines which were fashionable one day and forgotten the next. One man, however, must be remembered in this connection; his work still continues to be strongly active to this day and, in contrast to the other movements, still enjoys a considerable following: Samuel Hahnemann, the founder of homeopathy. Hahnemann was born in Meissen in 1755. At first he had little success as a practical doctor. Inspired by experiments with cinchona bark – which, according to earlier reports was said to have the same physical effect as malaria – he hit on the idea of diluting medicines since, in his opinion, big doses of a drug always began by making the disease worse. This sometimes went so far that the customary dosage could cause another disease on top of the first.

However, infinitesimal amounts of those substances which produced the same symptoms as those characteristic of the disease to be cured, formed the ideal medicine for that disease. For the disease was nothing but a 'depression of the life force' and a reversal could be achieved by use of homeopathic medicines. Hahnemann, who like Mesmer and Gall also went to Paris, summed up in an aphorism his belief in the healing power of weak dilutions of those substances which provoke the same symptoms as the disease they are used to cure: *Similia similibus curantum* (like heals like). Hahnemann's train of thought must be understood in the context of the era in which he lived. At a time when extremely drastic remedies were customary – under which many a patient died – such as repeated bleeding even to death, continual purging, induced vomiting, enormous doses of medicines which sometimes had a poisonous effect, and others, Hahnemann's system introduced into medical science a less negative emphasis than many of the forceful cures taught at the universities.

When Hahnemann published his *Organon* in 1815, an immense controversy arose, which neither the 'allopaths' on the one hand, nor the 'homeopaths' on the other, carried on in a dignified manner. It was just this difference of opinion, however, which brought Hahnemann's name to everyone's lips, acquired him countless followers and made it possible for him to conduct a profitable practice in Leipzig. When Hahnemann was seventy-five years old, the faithful wife he had married forty-eight years earlier died. However, when he was eighty, this unusual man was married again to a Frenchwoman, Marie Melanie d'Hervilly, who was forty-five years his junior. He moved to Paris with her and there quickly acquired a large circle of patients. He died, a wealthy man, in 1843 when he was eighty-eight years old.

Today, homeopathy and allopathy live peacefully side by side. It is obvious that practical medicine cannot carry out homeopathic principles to the last letter. It would not be possible to anaesthetize a patient for operation because the substances used in the narcotic cannot be administered in homeopathic doses. No local anaesthetic could be administered because doses of anaesthetic many thousand times stronger are needed than are commensurate with homeopathic conceptions. The pains of a hopeless case of cancer could not be alleviated by a morphine injection because the necessary dosage would not be at all homeopathic. Indeed, according to strict homeopathic principles not even a headache or toothache pill is allowed. That is why many doctors take from homeopathy as well as from allopathy whatever is likely to benefit their patients most.

The many different doctrines, to which quite a number could be added, demonstrates vividly the disruption of medical science at the turn of the nineteenth century. People theorized, speculated, philosophized, wrote books, established doctrines and, in Germany, under the influence of Schelling's nature philosophy, believed they could solve the problems of medicine by rational methods instead of using their eyes to look for facts.

Every individual principle was generalized; and all this meant that real considerations received short measure. Observation and experiment, the foundations of the further development of medicine were disastrously underrated; and it was only in the life's work of two German doctors, who lived during the first half of the nineteenth century, that a resistance to the all too theoretical attitudes of contemporary medicine was maintained. Their names were Johann Lukas Schönlein and Johannes Müller. However, before the attempts of these two German pioneers to direct medical science on to firm ground can be described, the further development of medicine in the other great German-speaking region, Austria, must be discussed.

30

*The new Viennese medical school. Karl
Rokitansky raises pathological anatomy to
a science made productive by clinical
medicine. Joseph Skoda publicizes
auscultation and percussion. Polypragmasy
and therapeutic nihilism. Franz Hebra
reforms dermatology. Ignaz Philipp
Semmelweis, the 'saviour of mothers'.*

The Viennese medical school
which, through the work of Gerard van Swieten and Anton de
Haen, under the wise leadership of Maria Theresa, made such
promising advances, had, a bare half-century later, already lost
ground again. It was not until the Paris clinic had long since
started on its brilliant, triumphal course, that a new wind also
began to blow through the Viennese medical faculty during the
1840s. The man who brought about this change was a professor
of pathological anatomy, Karl Rokitansky by name. Rokitansky,
who was born in 1804 in Königgrätz, worked under especially
favourable conditions in that clinical and pathological anatomy
had, for the first time, been firmly separated in Vienna. While, in
the other great centres of medical development – for example,
Paris – the clinicians were accustomed to doing the dissections
themselves, in Vienna, pathological anatomy had been raised in
status to a separate discipline, so a colossal amount of 'material'
passed through Rokitansky's hands.

This separation can justly be regarded as the cradle of all the immensely productive specialization in research in the future. Rokitansky, who had at his disposal thousands of post-mortem results, could, in the best sense of the word, raise the status of pathological anatomy to that of a science fertilized by clinical medicine, and so lay the foundation for a realistic pathology free from all speculation. His three-volume handbook of pathological anatomy, in which Rokitansky arranged his material from an anatomical point of view, and which was published between 1842 and 1846, was soon so well known that students and doctors from many different lands came to Vienna to study under Rokitansky. The Swabian clinician, Karl August Wunderlich, who set down his impressions in a book: *Vienna and Paris; A Contribution to the History and Judgement of Medical Science in Germany and France*, wrote: 'New life had come into the Pathological-Anatomical Institute since Rokitansky had been at work there. Foreign doctors flocked there from year to year in ever-growing numbers; it was again possible to learn something in Vienna; there were things to see which had been sought for in vain in other places.'

In addition there were, at that time, other prominent people in Vienna who attracted visitors from abroad. Thus Joseph Skoda, who was appointed to the professorship of clinical medicine in 1846, enjoyed a considerable reputation, not only in Vienna, but also abroad. He was of humble birth; his father was a locksmith in Pilsen and his brother also worked as a locksmith in his father's workshop. Both brothers, however, obviously had the makings of greatness, for the locksmith constructed a world-famous enterprise, the Skoda Works, and Joseph became one of the most outstanding doctors of the new Viennese school. He had a special interest in French literature, had carefully studied the works of Corvisart and Laennec and revived, by his work, the discovery of percussion which had been made three-quarters of a century earlier by his fellow-countryman, Auenbrugger (see page 211). Thus Skoda became one of the most enthusiastic prophets of physical diagnostics which he revived and extended; his reputation was so great that his lectures were by no means only attended by medical students. Wunderlich, the clinician from Tübingen, of whom mention has already been made, reported that in Skoda's audience had been 'professors, imperial councillors and old practitioners, who really seemed animated by true desire to learn the secrets of auscultation and percussion'.

Like Samuel Hahnemann (see page 252), who had been born half a century earlier, Skoda was extremely sceptical of the polypragmasy practised in his time – the customary bleeding, which was sometimes continued until the patient died; the continual cupping and use of dangerous drugs. However, as so often happens in life – and especially in medical history – one extreme led to another. Polypragmasy turned into the therapeutic nihilism which Joseph Skoda describes: 'We can diagnose an illness, describe it and understand it, but we should not imagine we can influence it in any way . . .' an utterance which is only too fatally reminiscent of Molière's words in *The Hypochondriac*: 'Regarded from a philosophical point of view, there is, so far as I am concerned, no more farcical and ridiculous person than the one who imagines he can cure another.'

Dermatology also experienced a reformation in the Viennese medical school under the leadership of one of Skoda's pupils, Franz Hebra, whose name lives on in dermatological terminology. Skin diseases, a step-child of medical science, had for thousands of years been regarded as 'eruptions' of defective mixtures of liquids. Hebra now undertook the pioneering task of arranging them according to a pathological-anatomical viewpoint. Thus, he was the real founder of modern scientific dermatology.

One of his closest friends was the Austro-Hungarian Ignaz Philipp Semmelweis, an assistant at the obstetrical department of the Vienna General Hospital. He was destined to accomplish one of the most brilliant feats of medical genius of his century. However an evil fate ordained that he should not live to witness the recognition of his pioneering work, but that he should die tragically.

Ignaz Philipp Semmelweis was born in 1818, the son of a rich Budapest grocer. When he was nineteen, he entered Vienna University originally intending to study jurisprudence. However, he very soon recognized his true vocation and, without a moment's hesitation, changed course and enrolled himself in the medical faculty. In 1844, when he was twenty-six, he took the State medical examination and shortly afterwards was appointed an assistant in the obstetrics department of the Vienna General Hospital. The obstetrics department was divided into two lying-in clinics, which operated an alternating daily reception service. It soon occurred to the young doctor, who was as ambitious as he was talented, that in the clinical division in which medical students were receiving their obstetrical training, the mortality from the dreadful puerperal fever of women in childbed was five to ten times as great as in the other division.

Although at that time no one had any idea that this disease was due to a tiny, living micro-organism, Semmelweis was too critical a person to be satisfied with the nonsensical explanations put forward by the professors, viz – 'because of a wounded sense of shame, caused by the students examining the women in childbed, the latter's resistance to disease was reduced'. With the tenacity of mind which was characteristic of him, he determined to find out the cause of this terrible disease which killed so many people, and a singular chance gave him a lead. After Semmelweis had returned from a journey, he learnt, to his consternation, that Kolletschka, the lecturer in forensic medicine, who was a friend of his, had died during his absence. He had lost his life in a strange manner: during a post-mortem examination one of his students had carelessly cut Kolletschka's finger with a dissecting knife. As a result, the lecturer had contracted the blood-poisoning which had ended in his death . . .

Suddenly, the scales fell from Semmelweis's eyes. It was he and his students who were bringing the poison of the dreadful

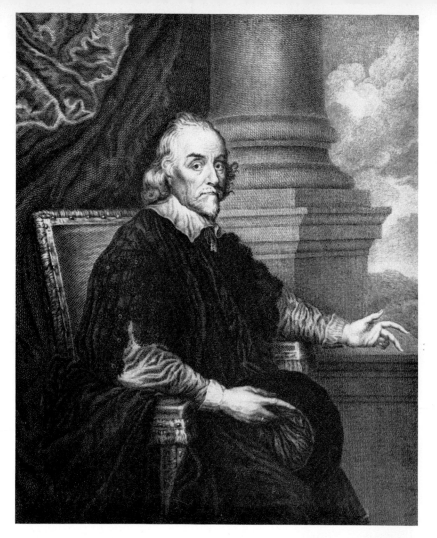

22. William Harvey (1578–
1657). Frontispiece by C.
Janssen to OPERA
OMNIA, 1766. From a
copy in the possession of
the *Royal College of
Physicians*, London

23. One of the first microscopes
invented by Leeuwenhoek
(1632–1723). *Staatsbibliothek
Berlin (Archiv Handke)*

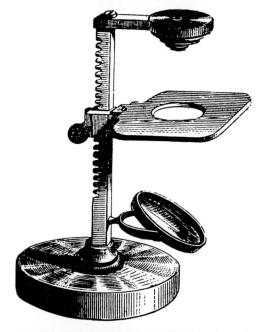

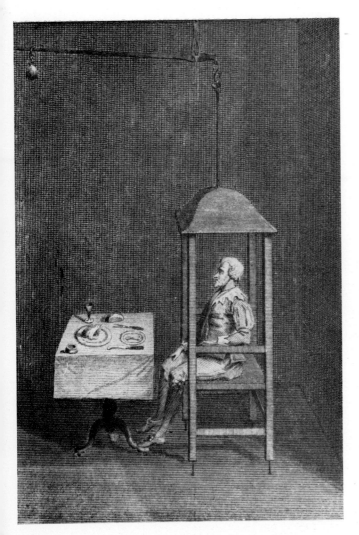

24. Sanctorius sitting in his balance. Engraving
by J. Beugo. *Royal College of Physicians*, London

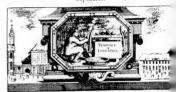

HERMANNI BOERHAAVE,
SERMO ACADEMICUS,
D E
COMPARANDO CERTO
IN PHYSICIS;
quem habuit in *[handwritten]*
ACADEMIA LUGDUNO-BATAVA,
quum
Octavo Februarii, Anno MDCCXV.
RECTORATUM ACADEMIAE
deponeret.

LUGDUNI BATAVORUM,
Apud PETRUM VANDER Aa, Bibliopol
MDCCXV.

25. Frontispiece from
Boerhaave's
COMPARANDO CERTO
IN PHYSICS. *British
Museum*, London

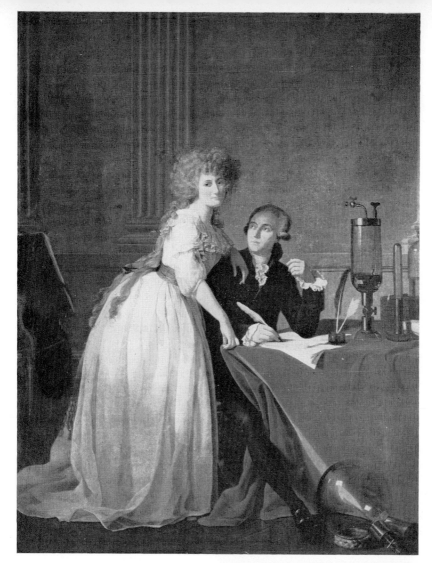

26. Portait of Lavoisier
with his wife. *Chemical
Society*, Burlington House,
London

27. John Hunter (1728–93),
by Sir Joshua Reynolds.
Engraving by G. H. Adcock.
Royal College of Physicians,
London

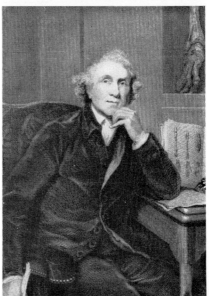

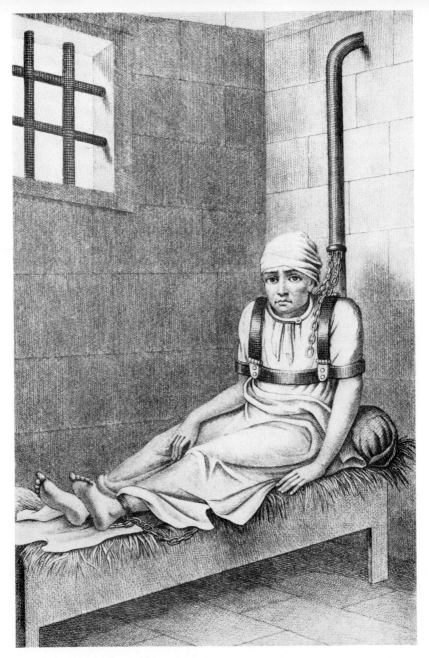

28. Insane woman under restraint in Bedlam. Illustration
in DES MALADIES MENTALES by E. Esquirol, from
a copy in the possession of the *British Museum*, London

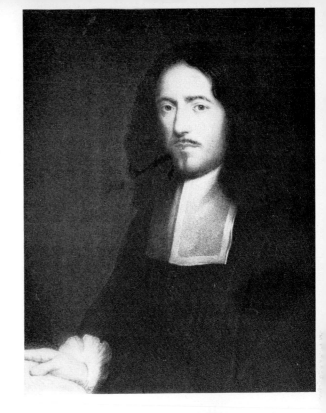

29. Marcello Malpighi
(1628–94). Portrait engraved
by J. Kip, from a copy of
OPERA OMNIA by
Malpighi in the possession
of the *Royal College of
Physicians*, London

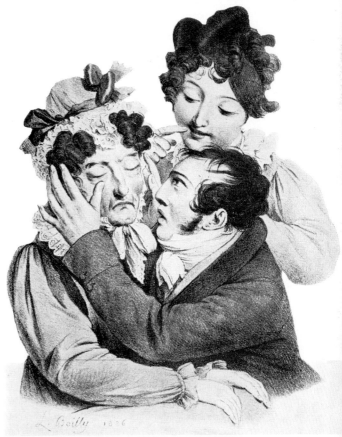

30. Mesmerism or animal
magnetism. Coloured
lithograph by Boilly 1826.
*Staatsbibliothek Berlin
(Archiv Handke)*

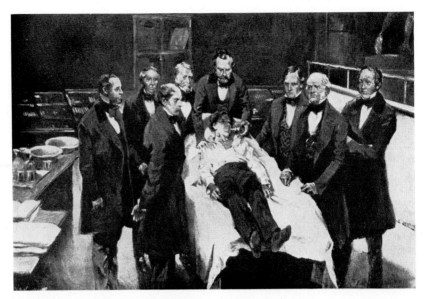

31. Apparatus for the inhalation of chloroform. Illustration taken from CIBA Zeitschrift No. 130/31.

32. Anti-septic operation with carbon-spray after Lister. Illustration taken from CIBA Zeitschrift No. 119. Both reproduced by kind permission of CIBA-GEIGY, Basel, Switzerland

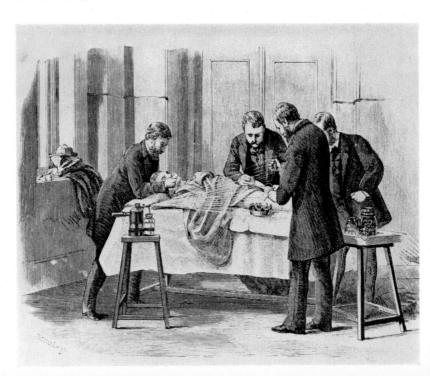

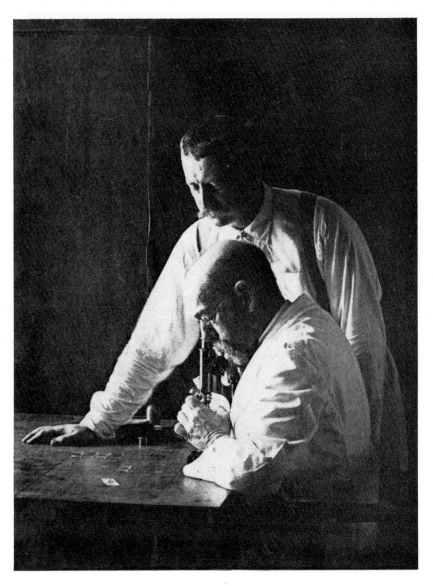

33 Robert Koch (1843–1910) in his laboratory. *Staatsarchiv Berlin (Archiv Handke)*

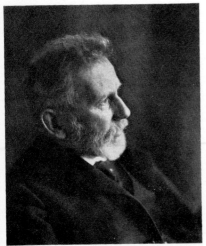

34. Paul Ehrlich. *Chemical Society*, Burlington House, London

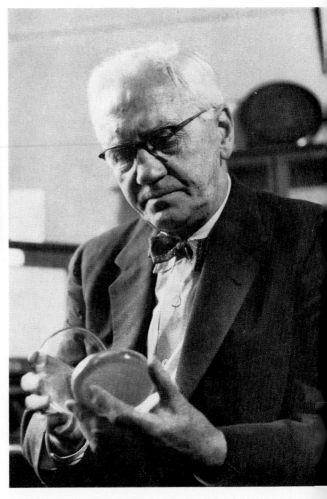

35. Alexander Fleming. From a portrait in the possession of *St Mary's Hospital*, Paddington, London

puerperal fever to the mothers; for, every morning, before he went on his rounds, he was in the mortuary demonstrating to his students, by means of dissections, the effects of the disease on the patients who had died!

Instantly, he ordered what to us today would seem obvious but in those days seemed revolutionary: that any one touching a mother in childbed must clean himself beforehand and wash his hands thoroughly in chlorinated water. Success was not long in coming: while in April 1846, in the clinic for which Semmelweis was responsible, eighteen out of a hundred mothers in childbed died of puerperal fever – after Semmelweis introduced washing in chlorinated water in May, the number of deaths in June was just over two and in July only one per hundred.

With passionate zeal he now openly accused the medical profession, and fanatically demanded that these measures which had proved themselves so successful should be introduced into all lying-in clinics.

With what success? What happened next reminds us of Goethe's words: 'We would rather admit our moral errors, mistakes and crimes than our scientific ones.' The embarrassing thirty-three-year-old assistant was dismissed by the College of Professors when his service contract expired.

Semmelweis tried to stifle his dreadful disappointment by throwing himself into experiments on animals. Joseph Skoda managed to push through modest official support for these experiments; Franz Hebra placed Semmelweis's discovery beside Jenner's variolation in the publications of the Viennese Medical Society. However, the influence of Klein, the head of the hospital in which Semmelweis had been employed, was still so great that Semmelweis's application for an appointment as private lecturer was rejected. It was only after the urgent persuasion of his friends that he submitted a second application to the faculty. A whole string of arguments took place; the great Rokitansky concluded them with the words: 'Semmelweis has a claim to the gratitude of the whole world.' The second application for the private lectureship was granted.

However, the appointment contained a spiteful clause: Semmelweis was not to be permitted to undertake any post-mortems during his teaching activities . . .

Semmelweis only stayed in this degrading situation for a few days; then he resigned his post and returned to Budapest. He had hardly left Vienna, however, when the number of deaths from puerperal fever again shot up to its former level in the lying-in clinic.

At Budapest University he was raised to the status of professor and had to start all over again fighting the same desperate battle against obstinacy, indolence and convenience that he had fought in Vienna. He felt that his work was declining into oblivion so he set down all he had discovered in a small book which was published in 1861. Its title: *The Causes, Concept and Prevention of Puerperal Fever.*

Then, however, his mind began to become deranged. His attacks against the doctors who did not approve of his theories passed all bounds; he did not hesitate to describe his colleagues as murderers. His behaviour became more and more frightening, and he had to give up his work at the university. In the hope that he might recover in Vienna he was conveyed to the house of his friend Hebra; then, when his stay there became impossible, to Joseph Skoda's clinic.

However, the unrestrained fits of rage which seized Semmelweis, who was suffering from dementia paralytica, made necessary his transfer to a mental institute. Destiny was kind to him. It saved him from a slow death in mental darkness. A slight finger injury led to blood-poisoning; and two weeks after his admission to the mental institute there died, at the aged of forty-seven the man who is known to posterity as 'the saviour of mothers'.

To reflect on the life and work of Ignaz Philipp Semmelweis is to wonder why he never hit on the idea which now seems so obvious, that of examining under a microscope the pus produced by puerperal fever. Had not a German anatomy professor named Jacob Henle already published in 1840 a work entitled: *About the Miasmas and Contagions of the Miasmatic-Contagious Diseases?* Did Semmelweis not know this or did he not connect it with his purely intuitive recognition of the cause of puerperal fever? Were not the trains of thought of the Frenchman, Louis Pasteur, already in the offing? Had not, in Glasgow, a professor of surgery called Joseph Lister already drawn practical conclusions from it? True, Lister's antisepsis, and the asepsis which was later developed from it, would not have been enough to prepare the way for the feats of surgery of today. For this, a further medical achievement was necessary – that essential condition for the accomplishment of delicate operations, the elimination of pain.

In this field, too, the young Viennese medical school performed pioneering work. It was the Viennese surgeon, Franz Schuh, who, in 1847, was the first surgeon from the German-speaking countries to perform an operation under an ether anaesthetic and thus, though he did not introduce it into medical science as an invention of his own, he was the first to make use of the new process which the English had discovered in such curious circumstances.

3 1

*The elimination of pain during operations.
Nitrous oxide for dental operations, ether and
chloroform for major operations. Louis
Pasteur solves the riddle of zymosis, and
prophesies the existence of tiny living bacilli.
Joseph Lister introduces antiseptic methods of
surgery. Antisepsis and asepsis.*

In earlier times, before the pro-
cesses of pain-elimination had been discovered, when someone had
to go through an operation, his state of mind must have been very
much like that of a man awaiting torture or execution. The letter
written by a grateful patient to the inventor of chloroform is
eloquent on the subject:

Before the days of anaesthesia, a patient on the eve of his operation
felt like a criminal who had been condemned to death and was
now awaiting execution. He counted the days to the appointed
time. He counted the hours on this last day and listened for the
sound of the doctor's carriage. He anxiously followed his
progress ringing the bell, setting foot on the stairs, entering his
room, unpacking his instruments, saying a few serious words and
making his last preparations. Then it was all up with his self-
control. He rebelled against the necessity, insisted on being tied
or held, in order to deliver himself helpless to the dreaded
knife.

262

In fact it now seems almost inconceivable to us that people living in earlier centuries could endure having a limb amputated 'from their living bodies' and even, during this process, having a bone sawn through. True, doctors did sometimes try to give their patients immunity from pain before an operation. In the Vienna State Library there is a manuscript by the Roman doctor Dioscorides dating from the sixth century AD, in which there is a picture of the root of mandragora and an exact prescription how a pain-killing drink can be prepared from it for people 'who are to be cut or burnt'. However, much earlier still, as mentioned in Chapter 3, the Ancient Egyptians appear to have used hashish, and the Ancient Chinese, opium before operations to kill pain.

Strange to say, the humane practice of making insensitive those people who were about to undergo surgery was forgotten during the Middle Ages which, after all, was a time generally quite lavish in administering pain; perhaps it was also dangerous to have anything to do with 'magic potions'. Instead, substantially more brutal methods were then used to achieve the same ends. The people awaiting operation were made drunk, or they were gripped by the throat, which not only filled the patient with mortal terror, but also stopped the blood from reaching his brain and so made him unconscious for a while. In consequence, operations had to be carried out with extreme rapidity which naturally was hardly conducive to the accuracy of the surgery. An operation for urinary calculus, for example, could be carried out by a skilful surgeon in one minute, and sometimes even in forty-five seconds.

It was not until shortly before the middle of the nineteenth century that attempts were made to use humane methods to anaesthetize patients before a painful operation. Impetus for this was provided by experiences gained in England from amusements described as 'frolics'. During these social games, the intoxicating and hilarious gas, nitrous oxide – which was discovered by Sir Humphry Davy, he Cornish chemist born in 1778 – was used to befuddle the participants; as a result nitrous oxide was also known as laughing gas.

It had been clearly established during these 'frolics' that the narcosis induced by laughing gas also rendered the participants temporarily insensitive to pain. Then, in 1844, two American dentists, Dr Riggs and Dr Wells, tried on each other and on their patients the pain-killing properties of laughing gas during dental treatment and particularly during the extraction of teeth.

From this it was but a step to the search for anaesthetics which could be used prior to major surgical operations, for laughing gas proved to be too short-lived in its effect for use in such cases. Two years before the first use of laughing gas as an anaesthetic, an American, C. W. Long from Jefferson, Georgia, had in 1842 used ether during an operation for the removal of a neck tumour. However, because he was working in a remote district, his pioneering deed remained unknown. Then other American doctors from Boston, New England – Dr Jackson and Dr Morton – recognized in ether a new method of inducing anaesthesia. Thus was reached a memorable milestone in the history of medicine – on 16 October 1846, at the Massachusetts General Hospital in Boston, the first surgical operation under a full ether anaesthetic was performed by William Thomas Green Morton. Again, a year later, in November 1847, the Edinburgh gynaecologist, Sir James Young Simpson – the man to whom was written the letter quoted at the beginning of this chapter – made use of chloroform as an anaesthetic for the first time.

The elimination of pain during operations removed one of the chief obstacles to the progress of surgery. There was, however, one other factor which made every surgical attempt seem questionable and every operating technique, however significant and subtle, illusory: this factor was infection by traumatic fever and gangrene. For an operation wound to close up, smoothly healed, without suppurating – which we should now regard as a matter of course – hardly ever happened in those days. Almost without exception such wounds closed only after a period of suppuration, and the patient could think himself lucky if this was only restricted to the area of the operational injury and did not lead to general gangrene or blood-poisoning.

In those days no one had any idea that microscopically small living things caused the infection of the wound with such dangerous consequence; therefore wound-fever, erysipelas and 'hospital gangrene' were phenomena ever present in all surgical clinics. Fifty per cent, sometimes in particularly bad periods even eighty or ninety per cent, of all patients suffering from an injury or an operation were attacked by these dangerous infections, which frequently brought death to even the slightly injured. Thus, even the greatest surgical skill was often in vain and, in the case of amputations, for example, scarcely half normally survived.

The suspicion that tiny living organisms might be responsible for the suppuration, the gangrene, the erysipelas, etc., was first voiced, albeit in a roundabout way, by the great Frenchman Louis Pasteur – born in 1822, the son of a tanner in Dôle, Burgundy – who, by his genius, brought about the start of the age of microbiology. According to the medical historian Erwin H. Ackerknecht, this represents the most important event in the medical history of the nineteenth century, and perhaps of all times. Pasteur should actually have been a schoolteacher; but, during his training in Paris, he heard a colleague of the famous chemist, Dumas, and at once the prospective teacher knew that for him only one profession was possible: that of chemist.

Very quickly he showed that he had made the right choice: natural talent and untiring industry, ambition and an unbending, pugnacious will to succeed, helped the young man to make his first important discovery when he was only twenty-six; it was to become, incidentally, the starting-point for an entirely new branch of chemical science: stereochemistry.

In spite of his youth, Louis Pasteur became a university professor in 1849 and then began a career of singular productivity, a life of research that was to keep the world breathless with forty years of ever new discoveries.

The young professor of chemistry's first scientific feat was to solve the age-old problem of zymosis. How does yeast change sugar into alcohol and carbon-dioxide? Pasteur answered this question with a series of brilliant experiments, during the course of which he also disproved the still prevalent belief in spontaneous generation; he demonstrated that microscopically small living creatures, tiny one-celled fungi – known as 'fission fungi' because of the way they multiplied by division – were the cause of every zymotic process.

Having acquired this knowledge, the inspired scientist at once extended its scope to other areas. As a result, he also succeeded in proving that the process of decomposition of flesh was also effected by tiny living fission fungi.

Now everyone took notice. Were there not a number of diseases in which the symptoms were very similar to the processes of decomposition? Did not gangrene and suppuration point in the same direction? Might not microbes again be involved? Might they not, indeed, play a prominent role in other diseases, particularly those of an infectious nature?

With bold inspiration Pasteur went on developing this train of thought, becoming more and more certain as he did so that the ever-present microbes, although they could carry out useful work in nature's economy, could also bring diseases and plagues, death and destruction to mankind. Since, as a result of his zymotic experiments, he discovered that each different type of fermentation was caused by one particular, and only one fermenting agent, so it was only a step to the assumption that each infectious disease must be produced by one particular, and only one tiny microscopic agent.

From then on Pasteur had only one aim, to unmask these minute enemies of mankind; he would probably have gone much further in his search for disease-producing microbes if a constantly recurring preoccupation with important practical matters had not drawn him away from the research of his choice. He saved the threatened French silk industry from destruction by identifying and combating the spotted disease which attacked the silkworms;

he occupied himself with the problem of weakened vaccines – which had been known since the days of Jenner's vaccination – and in doing so produced preventive measures against fowl-cholora, anthrax and swine erysipelas. His most popular discovery, however, was a vaccine against rabies, which he made from the dried spinal marrow of dogs suffering from hydrophobia.

When the indefatigable scientist was sixty-seven, his grateful fellow countrymen erected, in his honour, the famous Pasteur Institute which was to become a place of pilgrimage for microbe-hunters from all over the world. On 28 September 1895, the seventy-three-year-old Louis Pasteur died at his country estate near Versailles, laden with all the honours of this world, one of the most popular learned figures of his time.

Pasteur's prophetic conjecture that decomposition, suppuration and gangrene were processes which were in some way connected, fell on fruitful ground when it reached an English doctor named Joseph Lister. Born in 1827, the son of a wine-merchant of Upton in Essex, who, in his spare time, indulged a passion for natural science, Lister studied medicine in London, began his career as a surgeon in Edinburgh and, in 1861, when he was thirty-four, was appointed professor of surgery in Glasgow.

No sooner had Lister heard about Pasteur's experiments, than he resolved to find a method of caring for wounds which would eliminate the dreaded suppuration. It was a study of fractures which gave Lister the idea that provided the break-through. He asked himself why a simple fracture always healed cleanly whereas a compound one, i.e. a fracture which pierced the skin and often left the broken bone sticking out of the wound, was almost always accompanied by suppuration. It was not long before he realized that in the compound fractures the germs, which according to Pasteur's theories were everywhere present in the air, had caused the suppuration. Surely this assumption could also be extended to cover all other wounds whether they were accidental or brought about by surgical intervention.

Lister did not hesitate to draw practical conclusions from his deliberations. If it was the air which introduced germs into the wounds, then some way must be found to prevent the air from reaching them; moreover – the microbes themselves must be attacked with germ-killing preparations. At this moment the idea of antisepsis was born.

The most suitable chemical substance tested for this purpose proved to be a solution of carbolic acid. On 12 August 1865, Joseph Lister performed his first antiseptic operation; it inaugurated a new era in surgery. Everything which in any way came into contact with the surgical wound was rendered germ-free by being washed in a solution of carbolic acid; even the air in the operating theatre was sprayed with it.

The resulting success bore out Lister's theories; whereas, until then, suppuration and gangrene were rampant in his clinic as in all the others – the number of deaths from amputation was over fifty per cent – during the first three years after the introduction of 'antiseptic' measures, this number dropped to around fifteen per cent. After this, suppuration, gangrene and erysipelas became rarities.

Soon Lister's method found other adherents; but at first the English surgeon was not spared the fate of all scientific pioneers and originators of new ideas. People sought to belittle his success by rejecting and opposing his ideas; but at last Lister was able to see his work come to fine fruition. In 1877 he was appointed professor of clinical surgery in King's College, London; in 1884 Queen Victoria raised him to the peerage. It was then that Lister heard about Semmelweis's work and it says a great deal for Lister's high-mindedness that he did not take the credit for introducing the idea of antisepsis into surgical procedures but unreservedly acknowledged Semmelweis's prior claim.

In 1912, when he was eighty-five, Lister closed his eyes for ever and fate decreed that it should be a scientist from another country who completed the work which he had begun. It was left to the German surgeon, Ernst von Bergmann (1836–1907) a surgeon in four wars, to crown Lister's pioneering work by developing antisepsis into asepsis. From the process of germ-destruction he moved on to a method of working which was germ-free right from the start, as it is practised in all the clinics in the world today.

If we look back, it seems almost miraculous that all the great pacemakers in the fight against wound infections: Semmelweis, Pasteur, Lister and Bergmann, should have had no idea whether in fact there really were microbes which could bring about the inflammation of wounds and suppuration, let alone what they looked like. That this last veil obscuring the mystery of wound infection was finally torn aside was due to the achievement of a modest country doctor from the Harz Mountains, Robert Koch by name, who was just twenty-two years old when Lister performed his first antiseptic operation. Before his life and work are described, however, it will be necessary to glance at the general development of medicine during the nineteenth century and the fundamental progress made in physiology and pathological anatomy during this period.

32

The change from a mystical and idealistic contemplation of nature in Germany to a more critical and intellectual mode of thought. Johannes Müller directs German anatomical, physiological and medical research into a truer scientific attitude. Johann Lukas Schönlein also decides the direction which the development of natural science in German medical research is to take. First signs of the era of bacteriology.

W hile in Paris and Vienna medicine based on natural science was achieving considerable progress, in the Germany of the Romantic era the emphasis was still more on philosophy than natural science so, unavoidably, the history of medicine was influenced by this mental attitude. A fanciful and emotional life of phantasy, lacking commonsense and realism, seemed more important than a critical and rational view of nature; an idealistic way of looking at things was thought superior to observation, experience and experiment. A change in this state of affairs could only come about when the men, in whose hands the further development of medicine lay, had been converted from Romantics into accurate scientists. It is thanks to the fact that this transformation produced a number of outstanding doctors, who comparatively late in their careers turned to natural science, that Germany was to occupy an undisputed lead in the development of medical science during the second half of the nineteenth century.

The first of these doctors was Johannes Müller who – at first still under the spell of natural philosophy – devoted himself more and more to observation and experiment without, on the other hand, rejecting philosophy. Müller, who by his research and teaching activities stamped with his personality a whole age, was born in 1801, the son of a shoemaker in Koblenz, then under French rule. His teachers soon recognized the young man's unusual gifts and urged his father to let him study.

Thus, Müller attended the University of Bonn as a medical student where, when he was only eighteen, he was awarded a prize for a work on the respiration of the embryo. He graduated three years later and won a scholarship which enabled him to pursue a year's anatomical and physiological studies in Berlin. On his return to Bonn, when he was twenty-three, he became a private lecturer and two years later, reader. During this time he wrote a treatise on the physiology of the sense of sight; the twenty-five-year-old lecturer, who was strongly influenced by Goethe, sent it to the seventy-seven-year-old prince of poets with the following accompanying letter: 'I must leave it to your goodness and indulgence to look over most closely and correct this dedicatory present from a so-far silent and unknown pupil. I find such a close connection between what you have given us and what I have been able to develop that I am so bold as to make you responsible for all the consequences yourself ...'

In 1830, when he was twenty-nine, Johannes Müller became a professor in Bonn, and three years later he was appointed professor of anatomy, physiology and pathology at Germany's leading university in Berlin. This was the last time the three disciplines were to be united under one man; after Müller they were separately administered. However, in Johannes Müller there lived something of that happy versatility of past ages; he was an anatomist, physiologist, embryologist, pathologist, zoologist and palaeontologist all at the same time. Physiological and medical research is indebted to him for a vast number of individual additions; his immense work fills no less than a thousand printed pages containing hundreds of diagrams drawn by himself.

His work on the construction and function of the glands was epoch-making, as was that on the formation of the reproductive organs, the constituent parts of the blood, the spinal roots, the theory of tumours and many others. He incorporated all he learnt from the results of his experiments in his classic *Handbook of the Physiology of Man* which, for the first time since Albrecht Haller (see Chapter 22), discussed all questions of human physiology. However, as mentioned before, Müller's greatest achievement was that he changed a mystical, idealistic view of nature into a critical and rational natural science and directed German anatomical, physiological and medical research into truly scientific attitudes.

It was he who developed still further the experiments on animals and also the chemico-physical methods of examination, both of which were so vital to physiological and pathological research; he who also gave the microscope – which had been invented so long ago – its rightful place in the examination of healthy and of diseased tissue. Even Xavier Bichat – incredible as it may now seem – had invented his theory of membranes without a microscope.

Johannes Müller's reform of the methods of research meant that a number of outstanding scientists whose names will always be remembered in medical history, went forth from his Berlin school. A random selection includes the anatomist mentioned earlier, Jacob Henle; the co-founder of histology, Theodor Schwann (see Chapter 28); the inventor of the ophthalmoscope, Hermann Helmholtz; the evolutionist, Ernst Haeckel; and last but not least, the world-famous pathologist, Rudolf Virchow.

In spite of his brilliant position, in spite of his appreciative students, in spite of the recognition which was granted him on all sides, Johannes Müller was not a happy man. Evidently he did not succeed in coming to terms with the conflict between the remainder of his inherited mystical-philosophical attitudes and his work which was based on an accurate foundation of natural science. He was and remained a 'vitalist' – the only difference being that he called his life-force 'energy'. Everything organic was imbued with this energy; it directed the activities of life without being identical to them.

Müller never resolved this inner conflict; and this may have been why, in later years, he turned more to comparative anatomy and zoological studies than to solving physiological problems. His end was tragic. The outbreak of the revolution in 1848 shattered this wholly unpolitical man by forcing him to take sides and preventing him from continuing his scientific work. Worse still, he was visited by disaster on his way to Norway on one of his many educational trips in search of ocean fauna. He was shipwrecked and only rescued from the sea in the nick of time, while an assistant was drowned. Johannes Müller never fully recovered from this shock; a few years later he died suddenly in his fifty-seventh year. No one knows the cause of his death; he expressly forbade a post-mortem.

In 1824, the same year that Johannes Müller was working in Bonn as a private lecturer, a medical man, eight years his senior, Johann Lukas Schönlein, was granted the professorship of special pathology and therapy at the University of Würzburg. Schönlein also originally came from the Romantic school of natural philosophy with its positively confused ideas about the nature of disease; but he, too, very quickly adopted the methods of natural science. Driven out of Würzburg by political unrest, he accepted an invitation to join the newly founded medical faculty in Zürich, where his name is still honoured to this day. When the Prussians handed over to him the management of the Berlin clinic, he developed to the limit his extraordinary gift for the practical, for diagnosis and therapy; he introduced auscultation and percussion, microscopology and laboratory methods of chemico-physical examinations and held his brilliant lectures in the German language.

It was he who, in fact, really began the age of bacteriology which had already been heralded by various events; while he was still in Zürich, he discovered that a threadlike fungus caused

273

eczema capitis; it still bears his name to this day. Schönlein quite deliberately called his school the natural history school. 'We are returning to those bases, those pillars, from which medicine originally came. It is our purpose to rely upon the nature books – to go in a natural historical direction. The natural sciences shall be our guide, and show us how to see things in order to learn from them, and then to convert them into action.'

Thus Johannes Müller and Johann Lukas Schönlein determined the course of development of German medical science; Müller more in the theoretical, Schönlein more in the practical field. The medical historian, Henry E. Sigerist, judged that Johannes Müller and Schönlein had laid the foundations from which the Berlin school was to rise. After their almost contemporaneous departure a new generation of men came to fill the leading positions.

For the time being, it is true, the Paris school was still in advance of all others. It owed this position not least to the first great representative of experimental physiology, François Magendie (mentioned in Chapter 25 as Claude Bernard's teacher). Magendie, who was born in 1783 and also worked as a clinician, was, as already mentioned, the sworn foe of all vitalis tendencies; his chief concern was to explain all aspects of life in terms of exact natural scientific processes and physiological, chemical and physical laws; so he collected, through biological and animal experiments, a vast number of individual findings. While doing so he was once heard to observe, almost angrily, that every time one thought one had found something new, it was later found to have been described by Albrecht Haller. Curiously enough, he denied the existence of the red corpuscles which Johannes Müller shortly afterwards rediscovered and which today any student can see under even the most primitive microscope.

A still greater influence on the development of medicine was exercised by his pupil and successor, Claude Bernard, whose work has also already been mentioned in Chapter 25. Claude Bernard's physiological school in Paris competed with that of Johannes Müller in Berlin, and his pioneering work in the development of medicine in France was just as important as the research work which Johannes Müller carried out in Germany to further the progress of physiology.

Eventually, however, the scales began to come down in Germany's favour due, chiefly, to the fact that Müller's methods had inspired a number of new medical research scientists. They were to carry on the master's work on their own account.

33

*Ernst Haeckel's 'biogenetic law'. Hermann
Helmholtz invents the ophthalmoscope.
Karl Ludwig creates the 'wave-writer'
or kymograph, and thus introduces graphic
methods into experimental physiology.
Rudolf Virchow, the founder of cellular
pathology.*

Among the medical students carrying the coffin at Johannes Müller's funeral in 1858 was twenty-four-year-old Ernst Haeckel. Johannes Müller had introduced him to the mysteries of ocean fauna during a trip to Heligoland. A few years later, Haeckel came across Darwin's *Origin of Species*. At once he was filled with enthusiasm, and resolved there and then to make the idea of evolution popular and, by means of new research and discoveries, to give it an even firmer basis. Thus, the man who had described Darwin as 'the Copernicus of the organic world' became the impulsive pathfinder for the latter's theory of evolution; the so-called basic law of biogenetics, which he added to it, is among the most important scientific theories of recent times. According to this, the development of the germ of a living organism is in fact an abbreviated repetition of the entire historical development of that organism as derived from its heredity and its frequently modified adaptations.

Both Darwin and Haeckel logically applied the idea of evolution and development to human beings as well – Haeckel in his *Natural Story of Creation* which was published in 1868 and Darwin in his work *The Descent of Man* which was published shortly afterwards. In it Darwin wrote: 'If the Natural Story of Creation had appeared before I had written down my own work, then I would probably not have finished it. I find that almost all my conclusions are confirmed by Haeckel, whose knowledge is in many respects more complete than mine.'

As was only to be expected, the *Natural Story of Creation* and the *The Descent of Man* both evoked powerful and violent opposition and a cheap catch-phrase was coined to ridicule the originators of the theory of evolution, namely that they maintained that man was descended from the apes. Neither Darwin nor Haeckel had ever maintained any such thing. What the theory of evolution taught was that all living creatures sprang from a common root; whatever influences may have conditioned its later development, Ernst Haeckel's basic law of biogenetics was and remains an idea of genius.

Another of Johannes Müller's pupils, Hermann Helmholtz by name, helped to advance the development of physiology by exploring – chiefly with physical aids – the way in which the sense organs function and created the fundamental principles of the science acoustics. Helmholtz, who was born in Potzdam in 1821, the son of a secondary school teacher, really wanted to become a scientist and, in particular, a physicist. However, his father was a practical man who did not want to let his son study for such an unremunerative occupation, not having the means to support him as a private lecturer indefinitely. It was therefore decided that Hermann should study for something practical and become a doctor. However, his parents found it hard to pay for even this course of study, so his education began at the Pépinière in Berlin – that military academy where young people of good family could acquire, almost free, a medical training in return for a certain period of service as a military doctor.

Helmholtz took his state examination in medicine there and, in the thesis for his degree, he already demonstrated his interest in the nervous organs; he graduated in 1842 when he was twenty-two with a work on the construction of the nervous system in invertebrate animals – in the same year that Robert Mayer, the doctor from Heilbronn, first published his epoch-making ideas about the preservation of energy and matter.

At one time a professor of anatomy, at another a teacher of physiology, Helmholtz worked in Königsberg, Bonn and Heidelberg. It was then, while he was devoting himself chiefly to the physiology of the sense organs, that Helmholtz enjoyed his most productive period of research. At that time he also published his two basic works which are still valid in this field: the *Handbook of Physiological Optics* and the *Theory of Sound Perception*. In these he proved himself an experienced experimenter who enlisted the aid of all the resources of scientific research, all the laws of physics and mathematics, in order to discover the active mechanism of the sense organs he was examining, especially the eyes and ears. Moreover during his days as a teacher of physiology in Königsberg, he succeeded in making another revolutionary discovery which can be ranked as a pioneering feat and which has made his name famous: the invention of the ophthalmoscope.

The many discoveries and results of research brought the German school of medicine international fame; particularly so as a result of the physiological training establishment which Karl Ludwig (born in 1816 in Witzenhausen) had been running in Leipzig since 1865 – an establishment which was the equal of Johannes Müller's in Berlin. Karl Ludwig was also one of the real pioneers of medical development: his particular interests were the heart and the circulation of the blood, and he invented the kymograph with which continuous curves could be drawn on a rotating strip of paper. With this instrument he created the graphic method without which modern experimental physiology – and indeed all scientific and biological research – cannot now be imagined. Many foreign pupils, of whom many were Americans, flocked to him.

Meanwhile, however, a far brighter star had appeared in the firmament of German medical research. He was endowed with such brilliance that his light outshone even the famous medical schools of Vienna and Paris and, for a considerable time, made the German capital the focal point of pathology. Rudolf Virchow was the source of this far-reaching light; his medical fame during the second half of the nineteenth century can best be compared with that of Albrecht Haller which had extended throughout the whole civilized world a century earlier.

Rudolf Virchow was born on 13 October 1821 in Schivelbein, Pomerania, the only son of the local treasurer of the municipal council. He attended the secondary school in his home town and then, from 1839, studied medicine in Berlin where, in 1843, he graduated as a doctor. As a pupil of Johann Lukas Schönlein and, above all, Johannes Müller – in whose institute Theodor Schwann's discovery of animal cells had originated – he was soon enthralled with histology, an interest which was to have a decisive effect on his future work. As Virchow said: 'If the cells are the elementary constituents of the organism – its ultimate basic organized units in which the healthy signs of life occur – then the diseased, pathological processes must also have their seat in these same cells.'

For the time being, however, Virchow did not put forward this new pathological theory, but completed what was still missing from Schwann's theory concerning healthy cells. He corrected the earlier view by maintaining that cells are never created out of inanimate, formless matter, but constantly redevelop from other cells; crowning William Harvey's saying *'Omne animal ex ovo'* (Every living creature comes from an egg) with his own *'Omnis cellula e cellula'* (Every cell comes only from another cell). Thus it is Virchow whom we have to thank for the concept of the human organism as a 'cell-state'. This idea of the body as a social arrangement of individual parts, each enjoying equal rights with the others, was complementary to his exceptionally democratic philosophy of life. Rudolf Virchow also coined the phrase 'Medicine is a social science'.

Meanwhile the young doctor, who was as talented as he was belligerent and politically conscious, rapidly moved up the ladder of scholarly advancement. In rapid succession he became a surgeon's assistant, an assistant surgeon and then prosector at the Charité where he gathered such a vast amount of pathological experience that, in 1847, when he was only twenty-six, he founded a new medical journal of his own called *Archive of Pathological Anatomy and Physiology and of Clinical Medicine*. He gave it the following descriptive programmatic preface: 'The following view which we intend to take ... is the simple, scientific one.'

In the following year, the March Revolution of 1848 found Virchow active as a fervent and intrepid democratic fighter; the events of the time made him express extreme liberal views on the urgent medical reforms which were needed. His report on the typhus epidemic in Upper Silesia especially, was full of such unambiguous complaints against the authorities that, after the reactionaries had won in the spring of 1849, his services were dispensed with; he was only reappointed after innumerable applications and protests from his friends and from the medical societies – then only after a cut in salary and 'subject to cancellation at anytime'.

However, it was no longer necessary for a man of Rudolf Virchow's quality to live on charity. That same year the gentlemen of the medical faculty in Würzburg, who were more discerning than those in Berlin, appointed him professor in ordinary. Again at Würzburg, as a result of his untiring research, Virchow gathered a vast amount of pathological-anatomical material; he clarified the definitions of thrombosis and embolism and established the clinical picture of leukaemia, etc.

Meanwhile, it had begun to dawn on the Berlin faculty what a prominent scientist they had lost; in 1856 he was called back to the capital as professor in ordinary – better still, a pathological institute was built for him there and he was appointed its director. Two years later, his fundamental work was published: *Cellular Pathology and its Foundation in Physiological and Pathological Histology*. If Morgnani (Chapter 24) had recognized the organ as being the seat of disease, and Bichat (Chapter 27) the membrane – which, after all, was nothing more than a cell binding – Virchow now declared almost dogmatically that it was in the cell that the processes of disease took place.

As always, ideas have changed since Virchow's time. The present-day attitude towards Rudolf Virchow's cellular pathology, with its one-sided localized bias and its insistence on the disease being rooted in a certain 'organic spot', is that his theory does not do justice to the facts. The findings, not only in physics and chemistry during the bacteriological era which was already beginning in Virchow's day, but also of research into vitamins and hormones have, in the meantime, taught that a patient must be studied as a whole; they have revealed that his symptoms can well be discerned some way away from the actual organic 'seat' of the disease. Thus they led up to the present-day comprehensive approach to medicine. However, all this does not alter the fact that Rudolf Virchow can be regarded as one of the greatest doctors and medical pioneers Germany has ever produced for, as the previously mentioned medical historian, Sigerist, says: 'On his shoulders stands the whole structure of present-day pathology.'

Furthermore, in Rudolf Virchow there was still something of the versatility of the great doctors and naturalists of previous centuries. He continued to occupy himself with social problems intensively and impulsively; he cared about public hygiene and drains, etc; he founded hospitals, asylums and convalescent homes; he travelled to the west coast of Norway in order to study leprosy there; then he embarked on some ethnological studies in the Caucasus. He took part in Schliemann's excavations and by his careful research helped to advance ethnography, anthropology and archaeology. Last, but not least, he again took an active and lively part in politics, making clear, incisive speeches first as a member of the Prussian House of Representatives, and later in the German Reichstag (Parliament).

Virchow went on working to a great age, indefatigably active in many different spheres. He was awarded every imaginable honour and, on his eightieth birthday, deputations came from countries all over the world to offer him their homage and congratulations. A year later, on 5 September 1902, the greatest scholar of the age went to his eternal rest, and Berliners aptly rechristened the new pathological institute 'The Emperor Virchow Memorial Church'.*

It has already been said that Rudolf Virchow was a very belligerent man who opposed, generally with great scepticism, all innovations which did not originate with him. He carried on a bitter quarrel in the pages of his journal with Carl August Wunderlich, the clinician, who has already been mentioned and who made popular the clinical thermometer and who felt that cellular pathology was too one-sided; when Virchow was only twenty-five he ruthlessly attacked the Viennese pathologist Rokitansky, a man seventeen years his senior (whose work was discussed in Chapter 30), because he felt Rokitansky's pathological theory was too greatly influenced by humoral pathology. He did not recognize Semmelweis's reasoning because – so he said – he himself had often enough examined women in childbed after performing dissections and yet had never lost a patient from puerperal fever; and when Robert Koch – as will be mentioned in the next chapter – presented his anthrax preparations to Virchow with a discoverer's natural, diffident pride, the 'medical pope' showered the unknown district physician from Wollstein with biting scorn. In a parliamentary debate with Bismarck, Virchow went so far that the Iron Chancellor sent him his seconds.

In spite of all this, Virchow was certainly no dry pedant, nor

* After the famous Berlin church: 'The Emperor Wilhelm Memorial Church'.

was he humourless though, it is true, his humour was always somewhat at the expense of others. When he was once called to the bedside of a very wealthy old woman and found the entire family waiting for his verdict in an ante-room, he told them: 'You must be prepared for the worst – your wealthy old aunt is going to get better.'

34

*Robert Koch explains the life history of
the anthrax virus and discovers the tubercle
bacillus. The patriarch of microbiology
introduces the era of scientific bacteriology
by means of the examination procedures
which he originated. Emil Behring founds
the serum treatment and clarifies the concept
of immunity.*

Certainly Rudolf Virchow was antagonistic towards many a new discovery in medical development – especially the assumption of the existence of miscroscopically small animate disease germs – but in spite of his aggressiveness the great scientist did not oppose just for the sake of it. Indeed, during the course of his scientific work Virchow had become very cautious in his attitude towards medical 'innovations'. Now, however, medical development overtook him. While Virchow's star was still high in the firmament of medical research, a new light appeared on the horizon. As it happens, it came from the work of a man whom, as mentioned in the previous chapter, Rudolf Virchow had sent away pretty brusquely; the name of this man was Robert Koch. When he was born in Clausthal, a pretty little village in the Harz Mountains, on 11 December 1843, the third of eleven sons in an old-established family of mining officials, nobody would have suspected that he would one day become one of the most respected and famous research scientists of his era.

Robert Koch's childhood passed uneventfully. He was by no means a model boy, but a good, average pupil, in whose nature two qualities soon began to show themselves: the one, a great love of nature and all its creatures, coupled with a steady penchant and subtle talent for observation; the other – clearly the result of a casual visit to Hamburg 'the gate to the world' – a burning desire to travel and a violent urge to visit distant places and people.

However, when he was twenty-two, and still only a raw disciple of Aesculapius, he became engaged to Emmy Fraatz who was three years his junior and the daughter of the general superintendent of Clausthal. This meant that he had to stay at home and earn a decent living.

Decent, yes, but not always entirely enjoyable, for now began a wandering life as everyone's doctor in one place after another: Langenhagen, Niemegk, Rakwitz; until at last he established himself a little more permanently in the Posnanian country town of Wollstein, as public health commissioner for the Bomst district. The path which led there had been paved with worries, privations and hard, exhausting work; it was the tragedy of this great man's life that the wife he had married with such enthusiastic love, neither then, during the adversity of his struggle for a living, nor later, during his remarkable rise as a research scientist, ever became the true helpmate he so deserved.

Thus, a frustrating and incurable rift began to appear in their marriage and, the wider it grew, the more Robert Koch's subconscious groped for other objects upon which to expend the inexhaustible riches of his inner life. He surrounded his daughter, Gertrude, with a positively fanatical fatherly love and when, after his promotion to the position of district physician, he experienced some slight relief from his crushing and banal daily routine, his innate character asserted itself; the irresistible urge to search out the truth awoke.

The ideas of Semmelweis, Lister and, above all, Pasteur assumed ever sharper outlines in his imagination. Even though such an all-powerful man of medicine as Rudolf Virchow now, as ever, sternly denied the existence of disease-bringing micro-organisms, Robert Koch permitted himself to hold a different opinion and he methodically went to work to give practical proof of the correctness of his view. Now began an unparalleled rise, which was to see the unknown district physician from the Posnanian country town swiftly set on high as one of the aristocrats of science.

First, Robert Koch explained the secrets of the life of the anthrax bacillus which a doctor from Wipperfurth, Aloysius Pollender, and a professor at the veterinary college in Dorpat, Dr Friedrich Brauell, had already glimpsed. As already mentioned in the previous chapter, this scientific feat only brought him scornful, wounding words from Rudolf Virchow. Next Robert Koch turned his attention to the suppuration of wounds and proved that this was caused by various animate microbes, again, a scientific feat. Even such an outstanding surgeon as Theodor Billroth – the friend of Johannes Brahms, an art-loving, single-minded and acutely self-critical man, whose methods of performing stomach surgery still bear his name to this day – revealed in his book on wound suppuration, published in 1862, that he was not clear in his mind whether or not this was really caused by animate organisms.

It was not long before Koch, who had been called to the Imperial Public Health Administration in Berlin, embarked on research into tuberculosis. On 24 March 1882, with the modesty of a true genius, he was able to make known to a meeting of the Physiological Society in Berlin that he had found the consumption germ to be a rod-shaped fission-fungus which was between one-and-a-half and three-and-a-half thousandths of a millimetre long, and barely half a thousandth of a millimetre thick.

Now his fame could no longer be checked. There was widespread rejoicing; he was awarded honours and distinctions on all sides and became the most well-known and renowned scientist of his era. Robert Koch did not, as one might suppose, discover the germs of all contagious diseases; what he did achieve, however, by his tenacious, unflinching work was the creation of the initial procedures which made possible the construction of an original scientific bacteriology. By the ways which he had pioneered and signposted, he and his school were then able to find the cholera and typhus germs, the leprosy bacillus, the ray fungus, the erysipelas germ, the diphtheria and tetanus bacilli, the pneumonia germs, cerebro-spinal meningitis, plague, dysentry, the microbes of countless animal epidemics and many others.

While Robert Koch by a brilliant process of synthesis built the many individual discoveries into an entirely new science, he taught people to understand the nature of infectious diseases and epidemics and the manner in which they were transmitted. He also created weapons to prevent and check them, made clear – so vital for public health – why uncleanliness, dirt and disease are so closely connected, called into being a new public health service and so, by his work, introduced an entirely new era for all humanity.

Beside this gigantic lifework, he exhibited a humanity which, in its simplicity and greatness, worthily conformed with his outstanding scientific achievements. At the age of fifty Robert Koch stood at the peak of his fame; but he was still the modest, unassuming person he had been as a schoolboy, student and doctor. The entire civilized world overwhelmed him with honours on account of the health and happiness he had brought to people in every continent. As a result of his pioneering achievements international science regarded German research with great respect.

However, the man who had built up such a colossal achievement from the most modest beginnings was – alone! His marriage to a wife who had never understood him had finally come to an end; then a kindly dispensation of fate saved the solitary man from ending his days in bitterness and cynicism. Once again he was granted a great love. Robert Koch divorced his first wife and married Hedwig Freiberg, who was only eighteen, and whom he had met in the studio of a well-known portrait painter in Berlin. He never had cause to repent his decision for his second wife stood faithfully by his side for the rest of his life, the unfailing, intelligent, reliable and understanding companion of his remaining days.

At about that time yet another youthful dream came true, namely his never fulfilled longing for far-off lands, places and people. Now it became a marvellous, living reality. For almost fifteen years, accompanied by his beloved young wife, Robert Koch travelled all over the world – to the Orient and India, to Africa, the South Seas, America and Japan; heaping discovery upon discovery and, by his pioneering research, laying the foundation for the conquest of mankind's worst scourges.

He died after his return home on 27 May 1910, in Baden-Baden, when he was sixty-seven. All Germany mourned the passing of one of her greatest sons – science, the most successful research pioneer of all time; mankind, a benefactor and civilizer of international importance. On 30 May, two years after his death, the anniversary of the day on which he had announced his epoch-making discovery of the tubercle bacillus, the Institute for Infectious Diseases, of which he had been director, was renamed the Robert Koch Institute in honour of his memory.

Thus, his name lives on as one of the greatest research scientists of all times; also as that of an outstanding person in whom an indefatigable will to work, industry, thoroughness, accuracy, tenacity and singleness of purpose found its most brilliant expression. This is explained in the words with which, even during Koch's lifetime, Dr von Gossler, the minister of culture, honoured him in the German Reichstag: 'His powerful research work and his love of truth are only equalled by his unselfishness and humanity; and I believe our fatherland is fortunate to be able to call such a son her own.'

True, his otherwise so successful career contained one great disappointment: Robert Koch's hope that, from the tubercle bacillus he had discovered, he could produce a cure for that insidious national disease, consumption, proved to be unfounded, for the 'tuberculin' which was built up on this basis was a failure. However, even if Koch's tubercle bacillus could not be destroyed, could this, and other disease-bringing microbes, be attacked in some other way?

Reflections such as these were soon to occupy a young disciple of Aesculapius, Emil Behring by name, who was born on 11 March 1854 in Hansdorf, west Prussia, and who was the son of the local schoolteacher. As his parents were anything but wealthy, and young Emil had ten brothers and sisters, his childhood was not exactly rosy. The fact that he was able to study at all after leaving school was thanks to charitable patrons; he had scarcely finished his training as a medical doctor when Robert Koch had initiated the era of bacteriology, and Emil Behring immediately flung himself into the new and promising field of knowledge.

However, whilst the ambitions of his colleagues, who had chosen the same branch of science as himself, lay in discovering new microbes on the conveyer belt, so to speak, Behring was more drawn to the search for fresh methods of destroying them. He experimented chiefly with iodine compounds and even though his first attempts were not successful, they demonstrated such independence of thought that no less a person than Robert Koch himself became aware of the young scientist. He appointed Behring as an assistant in the Hygienic Institute in Berlin, which was at that time under his direction, and encouraged him to make experiments in an attempt to find a cure for diphtheria.

Behring now threw himself indefatigably into a series of experiments which were to have a totally unexpected result. The various iodine compounds were prepared, guinea-pigs injected with diphtheria bacilli and, when the infection had 'taken', the compounds were administered to the rodents. The bacilli were duly destroyed, but, unfortunately, in most cases so were the guinea-pigs. However, there were just a very few which had such tough constitutions that they not only survived the diphtheria but also Behring's iodine cure.

Energetically the young scientist went on working, but however many new compounds he tried, almost more guinea-pigs died as a result of his treatment than died without it. This bulk wastage resulted, one day, in a shortage of even such prolific rodents as these, so the guinea-pigs which had already survived both the diphtheria and the iodine were called upon once more. In order to try out a new compound they were again injected with fresh, active, diphtheria bacilli; but, strangely enough, the scientists waited in vain for signs of the infection to appear. The surprising thing became a fact: the guinea-pigs which had already been inoculated with diphtheria and which had survived the infection, did not become reinfected with diphtheria bacilli.

This was, of course, nothing basically new: that the survival of certain infectious diseases could render the organism immune from a second infection of the same disease for a certain length of time or even for ever, was ancient history; why, Edward Jenner's whole life work – the smallpox vaccination (see Chapter 26) was built on the basis of this fact.

What, however, was new was something else: it was the logical thought – what was the reason for this immunity? Where did it take root in the organism? Emil Behring, and the Japanese, Shibasaburo Kitazato – also a pupil of Robert Koch and also working at the Hygienic Institute – were the first to ask this question and to determine to solve the mystery by means of practical experiments. Now, suddenly, an entirely new sphere of work had appeared before him; with exactly the same eagerness with which he had previously searched for a chemical way of destroying bacilli, he now tried to discover the conditions governing immunity and draw the practical conclusions. From the start he was sure that this mysterious immunity could only be caused by some special condition of the blood and so he concluded that: if a single survival of the disease caused immunity against further infection by it, then the disease germs in the

blood must call into being a defensive substance which then continued to circulate with the blood, preventing the germs from a
second infection from thriving.

Having reached this conclusion, Emil Behring now had a flash
of inspiration: it must be possible to isolate the defensive substances which were called into being by the disease-bearing bacilli
and to make use of them in the fight against the disease . . . .

First, however, incontestible experiments had to be made to
establish that these ideas were no airy fantasies but were based
on well-founded fact. Therefore Behring took a little blood from
one of his cured guinea-pigs, mixed the serum with a suspension
of fresh, highly infectious diphtheria bacilli, and then injected
this mixture into a healthy, untreated guinea-pig. Behring's guess
proved right: the guinea-pig stayed healthy, for the added serum
from the immune animal ensured that the diphtheria bacilli could
not develop any further. At the same time, however, the control
test was carried out and a healthy guinea-pig injected with a
portion of the same diphtheria bacillus culture, but *without* add-
ing any blood serum from immune animals. As was to be expected, after the usual interval the guinea-pig perished as a
result of the characteristic symptoms of diphtheria.

The great experiment had been successful; that Emil Behring
was on the right road was confirmed when the Japanese Kitazato,
obtained the same result for tetanus that Behring had achieved for
diphtheria.

The German-Japanese co-operative work was crowned with
complete success. On 4 December 1890 an essay from 'The
Hygienic Institute of Privy Councillor Koch in Berlin' appeared
in the German medical weekly paper entitled 'Concerning the
Achievement of Diphtheria Immunity and Tetanus Immunity in
Animals' and the two research scientists, Dr Behring and Dr
Kitazato of Tokyo were the authors.

It opened with the following epoch-making comment: 'During
the studies upon which we have been engaged for some time past
into Diphtheria (Behring) and Tetanus (Kitazato), we have come

closer to the question of therapy and immunization in both diseases, and have succeeded both in healing infected animals and in giving such advance treatment to healthy ones that they later did not catch diphtheria (or tetanus as the case may be).

The whole world took notice: there was no doubt about it: the pioneering groundwork had been performed. However, would a way now also be found for the practical exploitation of the discovery? Would anyone succeed in making this mysterious substance, which was hostile to the diphtheria bacillus and circulated in the bloodstream of immunized animals, of practical use to suffering humanity?

With the unswerving consistency of true research scientists Emil Behring and his Japanese colleague proceeded further. Sheep were immunized and as soon as their bloodstream had become laden with antitoxin, blood was taken from the animals and the content of the serum tested on substances hostile to diphtheria. The gap was closed and Behring saw his work reach completion; for, if he injected the antitoxin which he had obtained from the sheep's blood into healthy guinea-pigs, then they could no longer be infected with diphtheria bacilli; and, further – guinea-pigs which were already seriously ill with the disease could overcome the illness with the help of the antitoxin.

The moment had now come for making the cautious transition from experiments on animals to use on humans. Fully conscious of his responsibility, Behring did not hesitate to take the step which would give mankind a weapon against the child-murdering infection of diphtheria. On 20 December 1891, in the children's ward of the University Clinic in Berlin, the first hopeless case of diphtheria was inoculated with Behring's serum; by the following day the condition of the little patient had already undergone a clear change for the better. Four days later, her parents were able to celebrate Christmas at the bedside of their convalescent daughter.

Once again a turning-point in the history of medicine had been reached, a new era had begun in the fight against infectious and contagious diseases; for with Behring's serum treatment a whole new branch of medicine had come into being. It was to develop into a vital, far-reaching department of science for, apart from diphtheria and tetanus, there proved to be a great number of other infectious diseases affecting humans and domestic animals, which could be both treated and prevented by the use of sera.

Behring, the pioneer of this achievement, was able to enjoy the rewards of his work. In 1895 he was appointed professor in ordinary and director of the Hygienic Institute in Marburg; in 1901 he received both the first Nobel Prize for Medicine and a hereditary title; in 1903 he was made a privy councillor with the title excellency. Fourteen years later, on 31 March 1817, he died at the early age of sixty-three and was laid to rest in a mausoleum in Marburg.

His gift to humanity is perhaps best described in a letter which his colleague, Wernicke, wrote to Behring two years before the latter's death, on the twenty-fifth anniversary of the invention of the diphtheria serum:

Full of gratitude and blessing, all humanity comes
before you today to honour and venerate the benefactor who
has saved the lives of so many millions of her children. We
all give praise for the good fortune which has enabled you
to experience this glorious day yourself, a reward for
untold effort, work, anxiety and cares. The will to triumph
helped you to overcome all difficulties, until this arch-enemy of
mankind had been defeated.

35

*The dramatic cholera experiment which
Max Pettenkofer, the hygienist from
Munich, made on himself. Ilya Mechnikov
discovers the phagocytes, and so explains
the nature of inflammation. Wilhelm
Konrad Röntgen discovers the X-rays named
after him. Karl Landsteiner isolates the
different blood groups and the 'rhesus factor'.*

Robert Koch had scarcely made
known his discovery of the tubercle bacillus when, only a year
later while in Alexandria, during a voyage of discovery to Egypt,
he also discovered the cholera germ. Nevertheless, time was to
show that the discovery of this dangerous microbe did not, by
any means, check the destructive disease for, as late as 1892,
it attacked the Hanseatic town of Hamburg – brought in via
Russia – and its unrestricted ravages claimed more than eight-and-
a-half thousand victims.

What was bound to strike the critical observer was the strange
and incomprehensible way in which the epidemic spread. Why
did the outbreak of cholera so conspicuously spare a particular
place – or even a district of a city – and, in spite of the fact that
no precautions were taken, did not infect the inhabitants of
those areas?

Could it be that the cholera vibriones, which Koch had discovered, were unable to trigger off a cholera epidemic by them-

selves? Were there other factors governing the start of a cholera epidemic such as, for example, the receptiveness of the person exposed to infection, plus some mysterious element in local conditions, determined by time and place, which might be found in the geological structure of the land or some other geographical influence?

Such questions as these excited the interest of Max Pettenkofer, the director of the Hygienic Institute at the Universiy of Munich. He was an unusual man, a highly original thinker, full of inspiration and successful in many different spheres.

Born on 3 December 1818 near Neuburg on the Danube, he was intended for a pharmaceutical career and was, therefore, apprenticed to his uncle, Franz Xaver Pettenkofer – who was chemist to the royal court in Munich. However, it was not long before he ran away from his uncle's apprenticeship – because of a box on the ear which he felt was undeserved – and went to Augsburg to become an actor.

All attempts to get him to return failed because of his pigheadedness; but it was unlikely that a man with such an inborn talent for research, could happily continue indefinitely as an actor. Pettenkofer soon abandoned his acting career and again devoted himself to science, attempting to study in two faculties at once. This time he made a clean sweep of both of them. In 1843, when he was twenty-five, he received certificates to practise both pharmacy and medicine.

With remarkable versatility and success, Pettenkofer immediately flung himself into every imaginable kind of physiological and chemical study. He invented a new procedure to establish the presence of arsenic, discovered the existence of creatinine (a product of metabolism whose appearance in the urine points to the presence of certain diseases), created the 'Pettenkofer procedure for discovering the presence of gallic acid in urine' and potassium thiocanate in the saliva, thought out a new procedure for manufacturing coloured glass, produced from wood a gas for illumination, showed the art historians how to preserve and renovate old oil-paintings, and a thousand things more.

When he was twenty-nine, Max Pettenkofer – whom his wounded uncle had prophesied would end in the gutter – was appointed professor of medical chemistry at the University of Munich; but his chief interest turned more and more upon the influence which a man's surroundings could exercise on his health.

After systematic investigation he determined the effect of the air, clothing, nourishment, water, soil, habitation, heating, ventilation, refuse disposal, etc., and so become, at one and the same time, the modern heir of Johann Peter Frank (see Chapter 26), and the founder of a new, rapidly developing branch of science: experimental hygiene. In 1865 he won recognition for his work, being granted the newly created professorship in hygiene at Munich.

He attributed special, enduring significance to the soil and ground-water, not just for the state of general health, but also for the spreading of infectious diseases and, when Robert Koch discovered the cholera vibrio,* Pettenkofer, who had been studying for many years the way in which this disease was spread, announced that, in addition to the vibrio discovered by Koch, another *local* susceptibility, connected with the soil and ground-water, must presumably exist in order to let a cholera epidemic spread.

However, at that time Pettenkofer's words were lost in the general clamour over bacilli, so the seventy-four-year-old scientist decided to prove, by a conclusive experiment on himself, that Koch's vibrio *alone* could not cause cholera.

It was already true that although, during that disastrous year, 1892, many people travelled to Munich from cholera-infested places, the Bavarian capital remained free of the disease. It seemed as if the mysterious factor, which according to Pettenkofer was necessary to create an epidemic, was missing.

He sent to the cholera-infested town of Hamburg for a fresh culture of the dreaded cholera bacilli, made sure that the microbes

* Scientific description of the cholera germ

were able to multiply in a specially adapted nutrient broth – so that in one cubic centimetre of the broth there were at least a thousand million germs – and, on 7 October 1892, to the horror of his students and before witnesses, the elderly professor swallowed this 'cholera potion' in one draught.

Pettenkofer went on living as usual, as if nothing had happened, and even swallowed some soda to neutralize the possible germicidal effect of the gastric acid. He ate in his usual hearty Bavarian manner, including stewed plums and drank many a glass of Bavarian beer and – to everyone's surprise – apart from a harmless attack of diarrhoea which he purposely left untreated and which disappeared of its own accord after a few days, he suffered no after-effects from this sensational experiment on himself.

Every one acclaimed the dauntless fighter who, by his fearless, self-sacrificing experiment, had prepared the way for a new era in bacteriology: the recognition that bacteria *alone* are not sufficient to cause an epidemic; that other circumstances must contribute to bring this about.

Max Pettenkofer was able to enjoy to the full public recognition of his pioneering achievement. After being raised to the nobility in 1883, he was appointed 'his excellency' conservator general of the Bavarian State Scientific Collections in 1896. He was also appointed president of the Bavarian Academy of Sciences.

On 10 February 1901, while suffering from an incurable disease, the eighty-three-year-old scientist voluntarily put an end to his life. He will always be remembered as an outstanding pioneer of medicine. That swallowing a cholera potion could also turn out badly was discovered by a Russian research scientist called Ilya Mechnikov. Although he started his career as a biologist, he contributed greatly to advancing the development of medicine – and, particularly, pathology.

Mechnikov was born on 16 May 1845 in Panassovka, in the province of Kharkov, the son of a remount officer. At an early age the lively, talented boy acquired an unusually strong interest in natural science and, by the time his older brother's tutor had finished acquainting him with the flora of Kharkov, it had been decided that he should become a biologist.

He studied physiology and biology in Kharkov, Giessen, Göttingen and Munich; investigated ocean fauna and comparative embryology at the biological stations in Heligoland and Naples and, when he was twenty-two, became professor extraordinary at the newly-founded university in Odessa. Appointed professor in ordinary as early as 1870, he continued working there, with interruptions, until 1882.

Then, having become financially independent after inheriting two estates, he and his family moved to Messina so that he could devote his whole time to the study of the wealth of ocean fauna around the Sicilian coast; and he was soon regarded as an authority in this field. However, he was not primarily interested in the systems of minor ocean fauna; his chief interest was in anatomical-physiological studies.

Mechnikov discovered the most primitive method of digestion to be the 'intracellular'* digestion of jellyfish and one day – after he had sent his whole family to the circus so that he could work undisturbed – when he was once again observing this process in the transparent creature under his microscope, he suddenly wondered whether there might not be similar flexible cells in the organisms of more highly developed animals, whose task was to provide, by ingestion and intracellular destruction, a defence mechanism against bacteria, foreign bodies, and other intruders.

By means of brilliant experiments, he proved that his assumption was correct and he devoted the rest of his life to its scientific establishment. Working with the Viennese zoologist, Clauss, he consolidated his theory and on this occasion he christened the migrating cells which perform the duty of sanitary police in the organism 'phagocytes',† that is to say 'devouring cells' because, by surrounding the invading bacteria, they either consume them

* A process taking place inside flexible cells
† From the Greek *phagein* – eating

and destroy them intracellularly, or they damage them by secretions and/or products of decay.

As a result of his discovery of phagocytes – which gave pathology the clue to the nature of inflammation and the constitution of pus – Mechnikov changed from being a biologist to a pathologist. Today, it is hard to understand why the Russian professor, who had such close ties with German science, should have received such a cool reception from Robert Koch in Berlin.

Thus, in 1833 he turned to Paris where Louis Pasteur welcomed him with open arms. Here, in the famous Pasteur Institute he passed the last twenty-eight years of his life, working in many and diverse branches of biology, anthropology and pathology and taking a lively part in exploring the questions raised by Pettenkofer concerning the comings and goings of epidemics and, in particular, of cholera. While doing so, he followed the example of the hygienist from Munich and swallowed cholera vibriones without becoming infected with the disease. However, when the same experiment was repeated by one of his pupils, it resulted in such a severe attack of cholera that his life was only saved with great difficulty.

In 1908 the deserving scientist – together with Paul Ehrlich, whose work will be described in the next chapter – won the Nobel Prize. In 1909 he gave a lecture in Stuttgart on human nature and medical science, which turned on the conclusion that man can correct nature's imperfections.

On 16 July 1916, when he was seventy-one, Ilya Mechnikov died of a heart disease at his place of work in the Pasteur Institute.

Mechnikov is a good example of how men who are not doctors can also be pioneers of medicine. This is demonstrated still more clearly by a physicist who quite literally brought into being a whole new era in medicine. That physicist was Wilhelm Konrad Röntgen.

He was born in 1845 in the Rhineland town of Lennep. He studied in Zürich, becoming a doctor in 1869; then he went to Würzburg and, in 1874, qualified in Strasbourg where, two years later, he was appointed professor extraordinary. In 1879 he became physics professor in ordinary in Giessen and, in 1888, he answered a summons to act in the same capacity at the Würzburg University. It was here that he made the phenomenal discovery which was to make his name known the world over.

A number of earlier German discoveries form, so to speak, the bricks out of which Röntgen created his achievement. In 1851 a Hanoverian mechanic, Ruhmkorff by name, had built the first induction coil. Another craftsman, the glassblower Geissler (born in 1815 in Igelshieb, Thuringia) extracted the air from glass tubes, filled them with different gases and then, by passing a high-tension electric current through them, made them emit coloured light. The service which these two simple craftsmen gave to science was so great that Ruhmkorff was awarded a considerable sum of money and Geissler, for the invention of the tubes named after him, was appointed an honorary doctor at the University of Bonn.

It was the German physicist, Hittorf, who first discovered the so-called cathode ray in Geissler's tube; his name, like that of the German physicist, Lenard, is closely bound up with the discovery of Röntgen's rays.

The exploration of the cathode rays was, at that time, a particular obsession of Röntgen's. One day in 1895, while he was experimenting with these rays in the Würzburg Physical Institute, he noticed that a sheet of paper, coated with barium platinumcyanide, which was lying on the table, lit up every time the electric current passed through the cathode tube. The most mysterious, curious thing about this phenomenon, however, was that the paper lit up even when the tube was inside a black box. The effect, therefore, could not have derived from the cathode rays; it must have been a type of ray hitherto unknown, of much greater penetrating power, which had caused the paper to become fluorescent.

Röntgen pursued his observation in a systematic manner. He examined the effect of the new rays on a photographic plate which had been put in a closed box and, during the course of the experiment, Kölliker, the anatomist from Würzburg, held his hand between the source of the rays and the plate. When the picture was developed it showed a clear picture of the skeleton of Kölliker's hand – the Röntgen rays had been discovered.

On 23 January 1896, with the modesty of a true researcher, Röntgen made known his discovery to a meeting of the Physical-Medical Society in Würzburg in a speech to which he gave the unpretentious title: 'Concerning A New Kind of Ray'. He called the new rays 'X-rays' and, as he did not make any copyright demands for his discovery, the Röntgen rays swiftly came into use for research and technical science throughout the civilized world.

Four years after his memorable speech, which had heralded in a new era in pathology and medical science, Röntgen was appointed professor in ordinary at the University of Munich and, a year later, he was awarded the Nobel Prize for Physics. He was still to make other important discoveries in his field before retiring in 1920. He died in 1923 when he was seventy-eight.

His work, however, will survive for as long as there is a medical science; for the Röntgen rays serve not only for the diagnosis of a disease but – after technical science had considerably refined their method of use – they also became an important weapon in combating many a serious disease and, in particular, malignant growths.

Only five years after Röntgen had made known his discovery of the X-rays, medical science in the German-speaking world chalked up a further triumph. In 1901 the Austrian serologist, Karl Landsteiner, discovered the blood groups – hereditary qualities in the blood, fixed in albumen-like substances (proteides) – which cause the blood corpuscles of one blood plasma to clot when in contact with those of another blood group.

For centuries past, blood transfusions had been made in cases of dangerous loss of blood (see page 175) – at first from animal to man, then, because of the frequent deaths which had resulted, from man to man. However, here too, more than half of all transfusions put the patient in mortal danger, and it was only after Landsteiner's discovery of the blood groups, which were compatible or incompatible with each other, that the blood transfusion which plays such an important role in accident-surgery today, has become a harmless measure.

Landsteiner, who later crowned his medical achievement by discovering the rhesus factor, was also awarded the Nobel Prize for his pioneering work in medical science.

36

*Paul Ehrlich discovers that the effect of
each medicine is determined by the
particular distribution of chemical substances in the organism. By creating
chemotherapy, he prepares the way for
the later victory over the pathogenous
micro-organisms.*

W hen the great excitement over
Robert Koch's and Emil Behring's work had begun to die down,
people realized that unfortunately by no means *all* infectious
diseases would respond to the serum treatment. In order to gain
ground in the fight against these other diseases, it was therefore
necessary to go back to the methods used by Behring when he
began his experiments, that is to say, to combat the microbes by
chemical means.

However, their use proved to involve almost insuperable difficulties. These difficulties were due to the fact that the chemical
compounds which were effective in destroying the germ almost
always developed an intensely toxic effect upon the organism
harbouring the germ. Therefore it was the task of science to
find substances which would destroy the disease-bearing microbes
without harming the host-organism.

The achievement of bringing about such a cure in the case of
syphilis, one of the worst scourges of mankind, belongs to Paul
Ehrlich. He was both a chemist and doctor of genius and, as a

result of his work, he became the founder of the modern science of chemotherapy which was to prove its success beyond all expectations.

Paul Ehrlich was born in Strehlen, a small Silesian town, on 14 March 1854, the son of the lottery-office-keeper, Ismar Ehrlich. Ten years later, he entered the St Mary Magdalene Gymnasium, a secondary school specializing in the humanities, in Breslau; in 1872 he passed his final examinations there and began to study natural science at the University of Breslau. He then registered as a student in the medical faculty at Strassburg, and found in the person of Waldeyer-Hertz, the anatomist, a sympathetic teacher and patron. It was also in Strassburg that Ehrlich came across a work on lead-poisoning that was to have an important effect on his whole future career as a scientist. In this work it was stated that, in lead-poisoning, the same organs or membranes which were, during life, most severely affected by the poison, would also, when dead – i.e. in the test-tube – absorb and store up in their cells most of the lead in a lead solution.

In a flash of insight Paul Ehrlich conceived the idea that certain organs or tissues in the body might have a special relationship or 'affinity' with certain chemicals and that this affinity is manifested by the attraction between the two. This idea was to continue to preoccupy the young chemist even though several detours had to be made before it could be translated into practical use. The question which interested Paul Ehrlich in this respect was that with regard to the varying capacities of the different cells and tissues to absorb dye. It is therefore hardly surprising that only a year after passing his medical state examination in Breslau in October 1877, he was in Leipzig delivering his doctor's thesis entitled *A Contribution towards the Theory and Practice of Histological Dying.*

For a candidate for the doctor's degree who was still only twenty-four, it was an immense and prodigiously bold work, which proved not only that he was already a distinguished medical man, but also, a chemist of unusual knowledge with an astonishingly creative talent, a talent which, in stating a problem, extended far beyond the technical science of dying. He arrived at the significant conclusion that certain parallels exist between the way in which the different tissues take dye and the effect of poison upon them; in other words, that the special distribution of chemical substances in the organism is the basis of every effect obtained from medicines.

Immediately after he had finished his examinations, Paul Ehrlich was appointed head physician at the First Medical Clinic at the Charité in Berlin – a very unusual distinction for so young a man – and here, too, he achieved several successes. Among other things, he introduced methylene-blue into the young science of bacteriology and, in so doing, produced the first general practical proof that there are dyes which will only take root in certain types of cell. If there are dyes which are specialized in this way, why should there not also be other chemical substances, i.e. those with medicinal properties, which would achieve an effect on one particular type of cell and not on others?

Ehrlich soon had an opportunity to give a practical demonstration of his discoveries concerning the way in which certain types of cell take dye: when Robert Koch on that memorable day, 24 March 1882, made known his discovery of the tubercle bacillus, Ehrlich left in the middle of the meeting and hurried to his laboratory. At once he began to make experiments with dye and by the next day was able to lay before a surprised and deeply impressed Koch, an ingenious and practicable procedure for dying the newly discovered tubercle bacillus. With minor alterations, this procedure is still used daily in thousands of laboratories and, as Robert Koch himself said, his dye method enabled medical science to obtain the full value from the discovery of the consumption germ.

It was not surprising, therefore, that the acutely perceptive Robert Koch recognized Paul Ehrlich's exceptional abilities and, in 1890, offered him an appointment at his Institute for Infectious Diseases and put a laboratory completely at his disposal.

Paul Ehrlich again achieved extraordinary successes in the fields of immunology and serology. He established his famous theory of lateral chains; and soon his name was so well known in scientific circles that in 1896 the co-operative ministerial director of Prussian universities, Friedrich Althoff, provided him with a work-place of his own in the Institute for Serum Research and Serum Examination in Steglitz. A year later, when Paul Ehrlich was forty-three, he became a privy councillor of medicine; and, in 1899, the city of Frankfurt-on-Main built the Institute for Experimental Therapy for him which later, as a result of a generous bequest, was enlarged by the addition of the Georg Speyer House for Chemotherapy.

Paul Ehrlich was now in a position to pursue his old never-forgotten ambition to look for chemical compounds – 'magic spheres' – which would only destroy disease germs, without doing any harm to the body cells.

Something he chanced to read channelled his work into a specific direction. He read that, at the Liverpool Tropical Institute, considerable success had been achieved against the trypanosomes – the so-called germs of African sleeping sickness – with an arsenic compound called atoxyl. Moreover, the German hygienist, Paul Uhlenhut, who was at that time director of the Bacteriological Institute belonging to the State Sanitary Board in Berlin, had discovered that this atoxyl was also extremely effective against the chicken-spirillosis germ which very closely resembled the spirochaetes of human syphilis. In addition, the bacteriologist and zoologist, Fritz Schaudinn, who had first discovered the syphilis microbes, had, immediately after their discovery, expressed the belief that spirochaetes and trypanosomes were closely related to each other.

Ideas began to take shape in Paul Ehrlich's brain: was it not possible to create organic arsenic compounds, similar to the atoxyl compound dangerous to man, which would, however, only destroy the spirochaetes or trypanosomes, while doing no harm to the human organism?

A further discovery by Uhlenhut proved useful to Ehrlich. In collaboration with the German research scientist Mulzer, Uhlenhut succeeded in injecting rabbits with the syphilis spirochaetes. Now, for the first time, the way lay clear for the creation of chemical compounds which would combine the most powerful destructive force against the spirochaetes without adverse effects upon the mammal's organism.

Using the services of an entire chemical and biological staff of collaborators, and by systematic and methodical work, Paul Ehrlich began to develop the ground for a new field of research. In retorts and test-tubes hundreds upon hundreds of chemical variations were built up and tested on animals whose blood contained massive quantities of spirochaetes.

The further they penetrated into these new research projects, the clearer it became that they were on the right lines: and, after more than six hundred preparations had been created in the chemical laboratory and tested by the biologists, they at last possessed a medicine which was both destructive to the syphilis spirochaetes and innocuous to the human body: Salvarsan.

On 2 September 1910, Paul Ehrlich – who had already been awarded the Nobel Prize for Medicine two years earlier – modestly announced his discovery at the 82nd Meeting of German Scientists and Doctors in Königsberg. His announcement created an immense stir throughout the then civilized world. Foreign governments bestowed high orders on Paul Ehrlich and scientific bodies and academies in countries all over the world invited him to visit them. During his visits to Holland, Denmark, Sweden, England and the United States, he had to report on his discovery and, in 1911, the German State granted him its highest honour – the title 'excellency'.

However, the restless and indefatigable scientist had perhaps demanded more of himself than any human being can give. On Christmas Day 1914, he suffered a stroke and on 20 August 1915, Paul Ehrlich died at the early age of sixty-one in Bad Homburg, where he had come in the hope of gathering strength for fresh work.

His full achievements for the good of mankind as a pioneer of medical science and founder of chemotherapy are to some extent only visible today. Working in directions which he indicated, German researchers discovered remedies for sleeping sickness – Germanin; malaria – Plasmochin and Atebrin; as well as numerous other chemico-therapeutic medicines. Even though the Salvarsan treatment of syphilis has been superseded today by the use of penicillin, it is nevertheless no exaggeration to say that, without Paul Ehrlich's work, there might not have been any sulfonamides, penicillin or other antibiotics; for it was he who taught the use of scientific research to create his 'magic spheres' and, by using such means in the fight against pathogenic micro-organisms, introduced a whole new era of medical science.

37

*The Dutch colonial doctor, Christiaan
Eijkman, introduces the era of research into
Vitamins A to T. Arnold Adolph Berthold,
physiologist from Göttingen, founds
experimental endocrinology by his
transplant of generative glands. Research
into vitamins and hormones directs doctors'
attention back to the totality of the patient.*

When Robert Koch, Emil Behring
and Paul Ehrlich were celebrating their triumphs, the excitement
engendered by the epoch-making feats of German research were
so widespread that what was discovered in other branches of
medicine received little attention. Yet development in the other
sectors of medicine had not stood still. Even before the turn of
the century, in 1897, the Dutch colonial doctor, Christiaan
Eijkman, had discovered the first vitamin – Vitamin B – while
studying beri-beri. He had observed that doves and hens which
ate an exclusive diet of husked rice – i.e. rice that had had the
layer of bran removed – suffered marked symptoms of disease
similar to beri-beri which, however, soon disappeared again if
the poultry food was augmented by the addition of bran.

Under the influence of the age of bacilli, beri-beri had until
then been regarded as one of the infectious diseases conditioned
by germs; however, Eijkman's observations established without a
shadow of doubt that food had some mysterious influence which

also played a determining role in the case of beri-beri, as it did in a number of other illnesses of so far undiscovered origin. Clearly, there was a gap in the science of nutrition – as worked out during the middle of the eighteenth century by Justus von Liebig and Karl von Voit – according to which the proteins, fats and carbo-hydrates, plus certain mineral salts and water, were enough to meet all the demands of the processes of life and growth.

It became ever more clear that a certain substance, until then unknown, must be included in order to maintain health. The guesses became more and more lively as to the nature of this mysterious substance which they encountered at first in maize, then in green fodder and root-crops, then in milk and then again in bran. In 1911, a little-known Polish biochemist called Kasimir Funk, gave this still quite hypothetical substance, which he believed was a chemically homogenous one, the name 'vitamin'. He had not the slightest idea that he was naming a concept of world-wide significance.

The first of the vitamins to have its constitution laid bare was the 'anti-neuritic'* supplementary substance in nutrition called Vitamin 'B', which Eijkman had conjectured was present in bran. For this discovery, Eijkman later received the Nobel Prize. The other classical vitamins were called A, C and D after the letters of the alphabet. Since then research into vitamins has resulted in the discovery of ever more vitamins and vitamin-type substances, reaching to the letter 'T'. Not a few disease conditions, whose causes had previously been wrapped in mystery, were explained as a result of research into vitamins, and treatment and/or preventive measures were made available: beri-beri, already mentioned; scurvy, rickets, hemeralopia or night blindness, certain nervous disorders and skin complaints, malignant or pernicious anaemia, and many other conditions detrimental to health.

A special position was occupied by rickets which, in days gone by, was particularly rampant among children belonging to the more underprivileged strata of society. Although it can be

* Directed against the inflammation of nerves

counted as one of the diseases genuinely caused by a vitamin deficiency, sunlight is needed in order to cure it. The factors involved in this complex relationship were only discovered in 1927 by the German biochemist, Adolf Eindaus and the American paediatrician, A. F. Hess. In the skin of both man and animals there are minute quantities of a substance called ergosterin. This is changed into active antirachitic Vitamin D by the ultra-violet rays in sunlight. A Nobel Prize was awarded for this discovery and this, plus the artificial manufacture of Vitamin D which soon followed, brought rickets under medical control – exactly 277 years after the publication of his monograph on the disease by the Englishman, Francis Glisson.

Although research on vitamins had begun during the last years of the nineteenth century, first intimations of a theory of interior secretions went back half a century or more. In 1830, Johannes Müller had already expressed the opinion that, apart from the known glands, there were others which secreted their fluids directly into the bloodstream rather than towards the exterior. In this way they exercised a formative influence on the different parts of the body during the course of the circulation – an echo of the natural philosophical era is still noticeable. However, the great physiologist had not supported his conjecture with experiments.

It was left to a physiologist from Göttingen to undertake these. He was Arnold Adolph Berthold, born in 1803, who was to become known as the founder of experimental endocrinology. In 1849 his pioneer-work appeared in the News of the Royal Society of Sciences in Göttingen. He had surgically removed the gonads of young cocks from their normal site and transplanted them on to the cocks' necks or backs. The result, as Berthold wrote, was that those animals which had undergone this treatment 'remained masculine as regards voice, reproductive urge, fighting spirit, growth of combs and wattles'; whereas it was well-known that the normal castrated cock (capon) could very quickly be distinguished from the uncastrated cocks in appearance and behaviour. Berthold concluded from this – quite correctly – that the general effect of the gonads could only be explained by the fact that they must produce a particular glandular substance which reaches the rest of the body via the bloodstream.

With the facts established by Berthold, the science of hormones, endocrinology, was born. For this phenomenon, the description 'interior secretions' was coined – as mentioned already in Chapter 25 – by that worthy French physiologist, Claude Bernard, when he stated in 1855: 'We assume that every single tissue and, in general, every single cell in the organism gives off products which pass into the blood and, by means of the blood, can exercise an influence on all other cells.'

One would have thought that this instructive assertion, plus the prophetic words of Johannes Müller and the practical proofs demonstrated by Berthold in his unequivocal experiments, would have become the prelude to a whole series of further experiments in the field of 'interior secretions'. However, for the time being, matters stayed on the plane of more theoretical speculation. True, the French neurologist, Pierre Marie, had found in 1886 that the disease acromegalia was caused by disturbances in the activity of the pituitary gland; and, during the same year, the Leipzig neurologist, Paul Möbius, declared that hyperthyroidism – a disease which had already been described as early as 1840 by a doctor from Merseburg, K. A. von Basedow – was caused by excessive activity of the thyroid gland.

Nevertheless exactly forty years were to pass, after the conclusion of Arnold Adolph Berthold's fundamental experiments, before the physiological and medical authorities realized that a new phase of thought on the workings of the vital functions had begun. It was 1889 when, at a meeting of the Biological Society in Paris, the French scientist, Charles Brown-Sequard, one of the most respected physiologists of his day, reported that after injecting an extract of animal testis into his own body he had experienced 'a radical change back to his former character of many years before; a surprising increase in physical strength and development of the intellectual functions; a stimulus to the appetite, regulation of intestinal activity and increase in intellectual capacity'.

Brown-Sequard's report became one of the most important landmarks in the development of modern physiology and medicine. The theory of endocrinology, which was already showing signs of progress had received its scientific authentication and, whereas Berthold's experiments had only enjoyed an extremely modest reaction, the echo of Brown-Sequard's report was now all the louder. Apart from the generative gland, the interior secretions of a number of other organs were recognized as, for example, among others, the pituitary gland or hypophysis, which had already been described by Pierre Marie as an organ of interior secretions; the thyroid gland; the parathyroid gland and the adrenal gland.

In Strassburg, during the same year in which Brown-Sequard had delivered his provocative lecture, two German clinicians, Von Mering and Minkowski, succeeded in discovering the basic connection between the pancreas and sugar metabolism. Three years later, Von Mering drew his conclusions from the experiments which he and Minkowski had performed. He caused diabetes in dogs by removing the pancreas, then replanted parts of the pancreas in various random places on the dog's body. The result was that the animals on which he was experimenting, lost their diabetes for a lengthy period of time.

Another year later, in 1893, a Frenchman, Laguesse, discovered that the mysterious substance which kept the process of sugar metabolism in balance was not formed from the entire pancreas but only from certain sections which were distributed like islands over the organ. Now a thesis was produced which a candidate for a doctorate, called Paul Langerhans, had worked out exactly twenty years before Von Mering and Minkowski had made their first experiments. In this thesis, dated 1869, these 'islands' were accurately described. Now it was confirmed that they were the places from which originated the substance which might well be successfully used in the fight against the widespread disease of diabetes. The first signs of the discovery of insulin had appeared on the horizon.

Shortly after the start of the new century, in 1901, Takamine of Japan obtained four grams of a crystalline substance from eight thousand bovine adrenal glands, which represented the pure, active substance of the adrenal medulla and was named adrenalin. Just three years later, the leading chemist, Friedrich Stolz, succeeded in the artificial manufacture of adrenalin, and so made the first synthesis of an active, internally secreting, glandular substance, independent of the organ from which it was produced in the body.

Meanwhile, now that more than half a century had passed since the birth of the science of internally secreting glands, the time had come to give the products of these glands a generally valid name. The act of baptism was performed in 1906 by two English physiologists, Bayliss and Starling. Since the internally secreting glandular substances acted as 'chemical messengers' which, through the activity of certain organs, developed a significant relationship with others, they named them 'hormones' after the Greek work *homaein* – driving, stimulating – and this description of the endocrinal glandular secretions has since become recognized as valid throughout the civilized world.

In 1908, six years before the First World War, Zuelzer, a research scientist from Berlin, was hot on the trail of the pancreatic 'island' hormone. He had obtained a substance from the 'islands' which, during experiments on animals, proved to have an excellent effect on diabetes.

After a further six years, the large-scale manufacture of this hormone was just about to begin when, in 1914 – the year when an American research scientist called Kendall succeeded in reproducing the crystallized thyroid-hormone thyroxin – the First World War broke out in Europe and Zuelzer had to stop work for the time being.

However, the world had scarcely recovered from the conflict

when, in 1922, in wealthy Canada, untouched by war, two young research scientists, Banting and Best, discovered insulin. At once their discovery conquered the whole civilized world and brought relief to millions upon millions of diabetics. Admittedly, it was only effective when injected, not when it was taken orally; and the fact that an American called Abel succeeded in fabricating a crystallized insulin four years later, in 1926, did not change matters. It was to be another thirty years or so before a treatment for diabetes in tablet form had been developed.

Two years before Abel had crystallized insulin, the American research scientist, Collip, had solved the mystery of the para-thyroid glands and, in 1924, isolated the pure hormone from the parathyroid glands of oxen. Shortly afterwards, during the second half of the twenties, two German research scientists, Ascheim and Zondek, discovered that the pituitary gland was 'superior to' the other glands having, so to speak, a commanding position. About the same time two Englishmen, Berger and Harrington, succeeded in creating an artificial synthesis of the thyroid hormone, thyroxin.

A new, extremely productive phase in hormone research began at the end of the 1920s. It was closely associated with the name of a German chemist and Nobel Prize winner, Adolf Butenandt. In 1929 this supreme German specialist in hormone chemistry succeeded in finding out about and producing artificially the hor-mone of the female generative gland – as did simultaneously and independently the American research scientist, Doisy – and then, two years later the synthesis of one of the two most important male hormones. In 1934 – the same year that the German re-search scientist, Holtz, discovered a substance 'A.T.10', which had exactly the same effect as the hormone of the parathyroid gland – Butenandt also discovered the structure of the female corpus luteum hormone and a year later a research scientist, Laqueur, from Amsterdam, constructed the other male hormone in crystal form and purified his synthesis.

This heralded a new era in hormone therapy – after all, it was

315

now possible to manufacture artificially as much of the most important hormones of the generative gland as people needed. The tentative testing of a treatment on animal organs, using an uncertain and varying quantity of the active substances, developed into a systematic hormone therapy with accurately weighed dosages; this has now given medicine a reliable weapon against many ailments caused by the deficient functioning of an internally secreting gland. However, what about when a gland secreting into the blood produces not too little, but too much of its specific active substance? The best-known complaint caused by the hyperactivity of an internally secreting gland is Basedow's disease, or exophthalmic goitre. This is caused by the unrestrained hyperactivity of the thyroid endocrine gland.

A chance observation directed the therapy of hormonic disturbances into entirely new channels. In 1943 an American research scientist called Astwood noticed that in guinea-pigs which were being kept for quite different experiments, the thyroid degenerated goitrously and, at the same time, its function became severely dulled if the animals were fed on an exclusive diet of cabbage or rape. Very soon the discovery was made that it was the sulphur-urea compound thiouracil which was causing the dulling of the thyroid; thus, the first chemotherapeutic substance for combating a hormonic disease had been found.

Another extremely significant period in hormone research began five years later, in 1948. Two Americans, a clinician called Hench and a chemist called Sarrett, discovered the adrenal hormone cortisone, and by this means developed a hormone-therapeutic treatment for rheumatic fever, diseases caused by hypersensitivity, asthma, etc. Shortly afterwards an American research scientist, John R. Mote, found the active substance produced by the pituitary gland which stimulates the adrenal cortex to produce cortisone.

However, the thyroid gland also held further surprises in store for research science. Everyone had believed that the problem of the thyroid hormone had been finally resolved by the thyroxin which the American Kendall had discovered in 1914 and which had been synthesized in 1926 by the two Englishmen, Harrington and Berger; but in 1952 English research scientists discovered a second thyroid hormone, named tri-iodthyronin. It also proved responsive to artificial synthesis, supplemented therapy with the active substances of the thyroid and, in several spheres, was five times more effective than the thyroxin which had been used before.

Meanwhile, efforts continued to be made to free diabetics from the irksome necessity of daily – or even several times daily – injections of insulin. Again, it was a chance observation which led to an entirely new way of combating diabetes. In 1955 German research scientists, who were testing a newly created compound in the sulfonamide group (see Chapter 38), discovered that this substance, which could be taken in tablet form without any loss of effect, possessed a powerfully reducing effect on the blood sugar. The first oral treatment for diabetes had been created thirty-three years after the discovery of insulin! True, the number of diabetics who were able to give up insulin injections in favour of the tablets was still small; but shortly afterwards, German chemico-pharmaceutical research found a new sulphongl-urea compound which enabled a greater number of diabetics, especially in the older age-groups, to change over from injections to taking tablets.

The seed which Arnold Adolph Berthold had sown more than a hundred and twenty years earlier, when, as a result of his experiments he was the first to discover the endocrinal function of glands and so laid the foundations of a new science, had in the meantime grown into a great tree, which, with its widespreading branches, overshadowed the whole development of modern medicine.

Both the vitamin research for which Christiaan Eijkman had prepared the way with his beri-beri studies, half a century after Berthold's experiments, and endocrinology have brought inestimable acquisitions to modern medical science. The present-day doctor's treatments cannot be imagined without the existence of vitamins and hormones. Moreover, both have helped to bring about the attitude under which, in contrast to the extremely local focus of the nineteenth century, doctors now keep their eye on the *whole* personality of their patients.

38

In an Elberfeld laboratory Gerhard Domagk
discovers the efficacy against spherobacteria
of certain pigments described as
'sulphonamides'. By creating penicillin,
Alexander Fleming, with Howard Walter
Florey and Ernst Boris Chain, opens a new
medical era.

As mentioned in Chapter 36 Paul Ehrlich – who was distinguished both as a research scientist and as a person and who, undeterred by a thousand failures, strode on with iron determination to the goal he had set himself – had become universally recognized as a benefactor of mankind in the best sense of the word. Nevertheless, as more experience was gained in the use of the chemotherapeutic measures he had devised, it became clear that most of the successes achieved by Ehrlich's chemotherapy lay against those diseases which had been caused by animal germs. The agents causing malaria are sporozoa; the tiny borers of sleeping sickness are flagellates as are, apparently, the spirochaeta of syphilis.

On the other hand, the treatment of bacterial diseases with chemical substances was a highly uncertain affair right up to the 1930s when the pioneering research done by German scientists produced a fundamental improvement. They then succeeded in winning ground in the fight against a number of the most dangerous, disease-producing microbes – the spherobacteria or cocci.

What that meant can only be realized by someone familiar with the dreadful conditions which were brought about by these blood-poisoning, pus-forming microbes – particularly in the days prior to the bacteriological era.

It began when Gerhard Domagk, working in a laboratory in Elberfeld, examined some pigments in the sulfonamide group to see if they had any special effect on bacteria. Domagk was born in 1895, the son of a simple village schoolteacher in Lagow, Brandenburg. He decided to study pathology, pharmacology and chemistry and, after he had finished his medical examinations, he worked as a university lecturer in Greifswald and later in Münster. After that he returned to Elberfeld as the head of the Institute of Experimental Pathology and Bacteriology.

Domagk had set his heart on doing the same for the plant-like, pathogenic micro-organisms or bacteria, as Paul Ehrlich had achieved with respect to the animal ones. His experiments with sulphonamides gave him the empirical fact that these pigments dye particularly colourfast, i.e. they enter into an indissoluble fusion with the textile fibres. Since bacterial bodies are essentially also cells, it did not seem impossible that sulphonamide might also form special relationships with bacteria.

In an extended series of experiments, a great number of different kinds of sulphonamide compounds were tested until finally, Domagk hit on a preparation that exercised a powerful effect on streptococci, for if a small amount of the sulphonamide compound was added to a test-tube containing a culture of streptococci, at once all growth of the bacteria ceased.

First, however, it was necessary to find out how this substance, which had proved so effective against a laboratory culture of bacteria, would be tolerated by a living organism. The biological experiments carried out on animals which had been artificially injected with streptococci turned out to be extremely promising. When, therefore, in 1935, people infected by streptococci were for the first time cautiously treated with sulphonamide compounds, the preparation proved just as effective as it was harmless in practical use.

Before long, the successes which were achieved with the new preparation exceeded all expectation; it was therefore hardly surprising that, in different laboratories all over the civilized world, a feverish search began for further sulphonamide compounds to combat the rest of the disease-bearing spherobacteria. Following Paul Ehrlich's example, the basic chemical molecule was altered and reconstructed again and again until the greatest possible destructive effect on bacteria, plus the most complete tolerance on the part of the human body, had been achieved.

Thus, a number of new sulphonamide compounds came into being, which introduced a new era of therapy in the field of infectious diseases caused by spherobacteria. The mortality rate for pneumonia, for example, fell from 30 per cent to 5–6 per cent; that in puerperal fever from more than 20 per cent to 4 per cent. Epidemic cerebro-spinal meningitis, which only a short time before had carried off half the patients in children's hospitals, as also infant erysipelas, which had a mortality rate of over 90 per cent both lost their worst terrors.

Domagk himself marvelled at the miracle which the bacteriological character of sulphonamides had revealed to him. Not long before his death, he said: 'If, a couple of centuries ago, a doctor had professed to cure an until then almost invariably mortal infectious disease, either he would have been locked up in a mad house or the cure would have been regarded as a biblical miracle. But we have become accustomed to accept as a matter of course the thousandfold miracle cures which the clinicians accomplish today.'

Gerhard Domagk had clearly overstrained his constitution with his unceasing research work; quite suddenly and unexpectedly he died of heart failure in 1963.

When Domagk was giving a lecture on his discovery to the Royal Society, London, in 1935, there was in the audience a silent, grey-haired man – fourteen years older than Domagk and an equally enthusiastic 'microbe-hunter' – his name was Alexander Fleming. He was born on 6 August 1881 in Lochfield Darvel, Scotland, and, being an enthusiastic disciple of Paul Ehrlich, turned his attention to bacteriology as soon as he had finished his medical studies.

In a memorial essay which he later published when he was seventy-two on the occasion of Paul Ehrlich's centenary, he wrote: 'Salvarsan was the beginning, a magnificent beginning, for bacteriological chemotherapy. I believe it was my experience with Salvarsan which first really awoke my interest in this branch of science; this experience, and the terrible sepsis which I was so often forced to see in soldiers wounded during the 1914–18 war. After my experiences in treating syphilis with Salvarsan, I wished I had some preparation which would attack the pus-forming microbes during my treatment of septic war-wounded.' This wish was only too understandable for Fleming had spent the First World War as a medical officer and, at the Military Hospital in Boulogne, had been a daily witness of the grim deaths caused by infected war wounds.

Alexander Fleming was therefore also anxious to find bactericidal substances and in 1928, seven years before Domagk's London lecture, one of those rare chances, which have occasionally brought about a fundamental change in the history of medicine, led him along an entirely new track. At that time Fleming was chief bacteriologist at St Mary's Hospital, Paddington. In the course of research on the growth and qualities of staphylococci, he had prepared a number of cultures in glass dishes, covered them with glass plates and then gone away for a short holiday. When he returned, the first thing he examined was the row of cultures and he discovered that the glass plate had slipped off one of the dishes. Mould fungus germs, such as are always present in the air of dusty rooms, had penetrated the staphylococcus culture and 'spoilt' it.

Fleming was just about to throw the dish away when, as luck would have it, he decided before doing so to give it a rather more thorough examination. This spontaneous inspiration was to lead to the most important medical discovery of this century.

What had happened? Alexander Fleming had made the significant and portentous observation that near those places where the mould fungi had penetrated the staphylococci, the latter had begun to dissolve. This could only be explained by the fact that the mould fungi produced a substance hostile to the pyogenic organism.

This discovery was not, it is true, as fundamentally new as it seemed at first sight. Thirty years before Fleming, a French military doctor called Ernst Duchesne had published a work entitled *The Antagonism between Mould Fungi and Bacteria*. The practical exploitation of this reciprocal effect is even older: in medieval times suppurating wounds were treated with mouldy bread and an English medical book of 1640 contains the advice to cover with mould wounds that will not heal. Finally, in the Balkans, a wound ointment is in use to this day which is prepared out of butter and mould fungi.

Alexander Fleming, although normally such a calm man, became highly excited over what he had seen. Could this spectacular antagonism between mould fungi and bacteria be exploited in the fight against infection?

At first, the work which was now begun – aimed at setting mould fungi against bacterial microbes – scarcely proved significant. Experiments were carried out with a fungus scientifically called 'Penicillium' and, even though the extracts which were obtained from it unquestionably contained a substance which could check the growth of disease-bringing bacteria – it was named 'Penicillin' as a result – this mysterious substance really proved far too unreliable. During every attempt to extract it in a pure and stable form from the cultures, it always lost its effectiveness. Therefore the experimenters resigned themselves to the fact that, because of its instability, penicillin could have no practical significance as a germ-killing preparation.

Then, ten years later, the Second World War broke out in

L 323

Europe and, while seeking effective germ-killing substances, the Oxford pathologist Dr Howard Walter Florey (who had been born in Australia) and a German biochemist, Dr Ernst Boris Chain, who had fled from Germany, again took up the research into penicillin.

This time the undertaking was crowned with spectacular success. Not only did they come closer to understanding the chemical nature of penicillin, but also to clearing up the reasons for its instability and therefore to finding a way of eliminating it. The result which proved most important of all for practical medical science, however, was the fact that penicillin is completely harmless to the organism and does not in any way damage the body's white blood corpuscles with their valuable powers of resistance. A further important fact which emerged from the increased number of experiments made with penicillin upon animals was that it was rapidly eliminated from the body with the urine, so that comparatively big doses had to be repeated at short intervals.

In 1940 matters had already advanced far enough for them to risk the transfer from laboratory experiments to use on actual patients. After numerous experiments had been made on animals a policeman in Oxford, who was suffering from an acute case of blood-poisoning caused by staphylococci, became the first human being to be treated with penicillin. After five days' application of the new remedy the outcome was obvious and the patient's eventual recovery could be hoped for. However there was only a very small store of the medicine and this was soon exhausted. The injections had to be stopped for a few days, the blood-poisoning returned, and the patient died.

Doctors now knew for certain that, in order to achieve its effect on humans, the organism must be kept under the constant control of penicillin for the length of time necessary to achieve a cure; this meant that it was necessary to give penicillin injections every two or three hours. The next attempt was not undertaken until a sufficient supply of penicillin was available. The patient was a boy with coxitis. He recovered.

As a result of these experiences, there was no longer any doubt that the new medicine had a future; but, as so often happens when new medicines are introduced, the step from the test-tube to mass-production in factories at first seemed to be surrounded by insurmountable difficulties.

These were not resolved until the United States took over the problem and invited the English research scientists to go to America and continue their experiments there. Supported by the rich resources of the U.S.A., work was begun with the utmost energy to find a method of producing large-scale quantities of penicillin.

Since the Second World War, a large number of lesser varieties of fungus have been examined for bactericidal qualities; the search for ever newer penicillin-type preparations, which were given the name 'antibiotics', is being actively pursued at the present time. Antibiotics possessing the most diverse therapeutic qualities, as well as semi-synthetic penicillins, are today being manufactured in many of the laboratories belonging to the chemico-pharmaceutical industry. Some of them have to be injected, others can be taken orally without any diminution of effect, and they can be used against almost all pathogenic micro-organisms with the exception of viruses – the discovery of which will be described in the next chapter. Meanwhile, the creation of penicillin has by no means rendered the previously discovered sulphona-amides superfluous. Both groups of medicines can be used most effectively in certain cases to complement each other.

Alexander Fleming, Howard Walter Florey and Ernst Boris Chain were awarded the Nobel Prize in 1945. The remarkable modesty of Fleming – whose work heralded a whole new era in medicine – is demonstrated by a statement he made shortly before his death from a heart-attack on 11 March 1955: 'Every-where I go people want to thank me for saving their lives. I really don't know why they do that. Nature created penicillin. I only found it.'

39

*The smallest of all mankind's enemies: the
viruses. The electron microscope turns the
ultra-microscopic into filtrable bacilli. At
the frontier of life and lifelessness. The fight
against virus diseases.*

Exactly ten years after Robert
Koch had discovered the tubercle bacillus, a Russian research
scientist named Ivanovski began a study of the 'mosaic' disease
which was causing such havoc to agriculture by its attacks on
tobacco, potatoes and tomatoes. Ivanovski, at the height of the
bacillus era, was convinced that the mosaic disease was caused by
bacteria and used every imaginable method in an attempt to get
the better of the disease-carrying organism. However, even the
most powerful microscope in use at that time was unable to
reveal the micro-organism which caused the 'mosaic' disease.

Therefore, the organism must be ultra-microscopic, i.e. beyond
visibility; in order to prove that it did in fact exist, Ivanovski
worked out an experiment which was the start of the history of
virus research. He made up a liquid from the cells of tobacco
plants which had been highly infected with mosaic disease, and
first passed it through a filter with pores so fine that even the
smallest germs then known would be trapped by it. Ivanovski
then treated healthy plants with this liquid which was now
certainly free of bacteria. The plants promptly became infected
with mosaic disease. The disease-bearing organism must therefore

be so small that it would remain invisible even under a microscope. It was given the name virus.

Shortly afterwards a number of infections attacking both man and animals were recognized as virus diseases; among others, haemorrhagic smallpox, acute poliomyelitis, rabies, measles, influenza, chicken-pox, German measles, herpes zoster, mumps, psittacosis, yellow fever, foot-and-mouth disease, fowl pest.

For another forty years the organisms causing these diseases were regarded as ultra-visible, or beyond visibility, until in 1932 two medical men, E. Paschen and E. Nauck, in the Institute for Marine and Tropical Diseases in Hamburg, succeeded in trapping the first virus (Paschen's bodies) under the miscroscope. As a result, the description ultra-visible was revised; the micro-organisms which passed through the bacteria-proof ultra-filter were thereafter known as filtrable disease-bearing organisms.

However, a further seven years were to pass before the tobacco mosaic virus gave up its secrets in 1939. The fact that virology then made progress previously imagined impossible was thanks to the electron microscope built by German research scientists and which, in contrast to the usual 'light' microscope, used electron rays instead of light rays. Because of the much shorter wave-length of these rays, the electron microscope – which, as a result of further discoveries was substantially improved by the engineer Professor E. Ruska in 1953 – possesses a disproportionately greater power than the light microscope. It achieves one hundred thousandfold magnifications and more and, with its help, it is possible to distinguish objects that are only a millionth of a millimetre apart. Modern virology, the research into heredity and the research of albumin molecules, would not have been conceivable without the electron microscope; this miracle of technical science has therefore decisively advanced the development of medicine.

Four years before it was made visible, the tobacco virus had already amazed the scientific world with a property unheard of in a living organism. In 1935 the American research scientist,

W. M. Stanley, working at the Rockefeller Institute in Princeton, U.S.A., succeeded in making a crystallized extract of the virus and keeping it infectious in that form. He could reduce the crystal to a solution as often as he liked and then let it crystallize again; its infectious qualities remained unaffected. This seemed to cause the frontier between living and lifeless substances to waver for, until then, nobody had believed in the possibility that living matter could persist in crystal form.

Meanwhile, the electron microscope had helped people to penetrate still further into the fine structure of the viruses. As a result it was shown that viruses – some of which are scarcely larger than big molecules – only consist, chemically, of two substances: namely, a greater part of albumen (protein) and a smaller part consisting of nucleinic acid. In this they correspond exactly with the units containing the hereditary factors known as 'genes' which are arranged in strings of germ cells called chromosomes.

At a meeting of the Society of German Natural Scientists and Doctors in 1958, Dr G. Schramm, professor of genetics at the Max Planck Institute for Virus Research in Tübingen, announced that he had succeeded in altering in certain ways the hereditary substance of viruses – which, of course, exactly correspond to those of genes. This achievement is but a step from the rather depressing idea that one day the hereditary substance in human beings can also be manipulated in order, for example, to strengthen certain tendencies and cause others to disappear. This possibility has recently come still closer as a result of a scientific feat performed by American research scientists at Stanford University in California under the direction of Nobel Prize winner, Arthur Kornberg, in December 1967. They succeeded in reproducing, in synthetic form, the substance carrying the hereditary factor and with it the genetic code of the living cell, and were therefore in a position to interfere with the transfer of hereditary influences.

Although it is true that such considerations still lie very much in the future, virology had already achieved very substantial and significant successes in the development of medical science. They can be valued the more highly as the virus bodies have proved extraordinarily difficult to combat. The reason for this is as follows: when bacteriological substances are attacked with preparations such as sulphonamides or antibiotics, their metabolism is damaged. Viruses, however, do not have metabolism; they can even be said to have no life of their own. Like some parasites, they 'borrow' it from the host cell. Therefore all measures against viruses must, in the last resort, also be directed against the host cell.

That is why, with few exceptions, once a virus infection has broken out a treatment can scarcely ever succeed. Virologists have therefore concentrated all the more on attempts to find effective protective measures against the most dangerous virus diseases. Thus, the American bacteriologist and serologist, Max Theiler (born in 1899) carried out research into the yellow fever virus and developed a yellow fever serum which took most of the terror from this disease which, in the past – especially in Central and South America, and Central and West Africa – had exacted so many victims. Theiler was awarded the Nobel Prize for Medicine for this scientific feat.

Of more recent date is the oral inoculation against poliomyelitis which is associated with the name of the American bacteriologist, Albert Bruce Sabin (born in 1906). Whereas, before the introduction of this inoculation, polio was horrifyingly on the increase, and attacking adults more and more frequently, since the introduction of the oral inoculation this has been reduced to a minimum.

Sera against other virus diseases have, in some cases, already been created and in others virologists are still working at their development. In any case, if virology continues at its present rate, progressive medical science will also give us weapons against the very smallest enemies of mankind.

40

Modern progress in the theory of mental disorders. Wilhelm Griesinger founds scientific psychiatry. Ivan Petrovich Pavlov and the theory of reflexes. Emil Kraepelin as a systematizer of psychoses. Julius Wagner-Jaurreg's principle 'disease against Disease'. Wilhelm Heinrich Erb and electrotherapy. Sigmund Freud and the birth of psychoanalysis. The 'spiritual medicines'.

Courageously standing alone, Philippe Pinel had freed the insane during the French Revolution (see Chapter 26); for the time being, however, this did not produce any fundamental change in the fate of the mental patients in other countries. Although hospitals for the treatment of mental patients were set up in other places too, it was to be several decades, in fact not until the second half of the nineteenth century, before the violent and brutal methods by which they were treated gave way to humane ones. Punishment with whips, sticks and switches, forced standing and turning-chairs, were still the 'treatments' meted out to both mentally deranged and raving patients.

It was not until natural science triumphed in Germany that a psychiatric science was created there. The man who may count as its founder was a Swabian doctor named Wilhelm Griesinger.

Born in Stuttgart in 1817, he made a special study of mental disorders when he was already enjoying a distinguished reputation as a resident clinician and, when he was sixty, became professor and leading physician at the mental hospital and neuropathic division of the Charité in Berlin.

Griesinger, whose work was completely in accordance with scientific, physiological and anti-Romantic medicine, sought the origin of mental diseases in cerebro-pathological changes and so conceived the psychoses as brain diseases. He was the first to connect the condition of the nerve substance with the mental processes. Although he made such valuable contributions to cerebro-pathological research, the future was to prove that by no means all mental illnesses are accompanied by a pathological anatomical condition of the brain.

The assumption that it is basically the physiological processes which underlie the functioning of the brain cells was proved by the pioneering experiments of a Russian physiologist, Ivan Petrovich Pavlov, the son of a priest, who was born in 1849 in Rjasan, south-east of Moscow. Pavlov, too, was intended for the Church, but he was so strongly drawn towards medicine that he managed to get his way and take up its study. However, he was less interested in practising medicine than in studying physiology. In doing so, Pavlov, who worked as assistant to Bernard in Paris and Carl Ludwig in Leipzig, not only brought the physiological knowledge of the West to Russia but also, after he had already caused a stir by a series of illuminating experiments on the digestion, brought into being an entirely new experimental physiology of the central nervous system. From Pavlov stems the recognition that 'absolute', empirically taught reflexes are located in the much younger, from an evolutionary view, cerebral cortex.

Pavlov had already been awarded the Nobel Prize in 1904. Every imaginable honour was given him at the International Physiological Congress in Leningrad in 1935; a year later, when he was eighty-six, he died. His discoveries were complemented by those of the physiologist, Walter Rudolf Hess, who was born in 1881 in Frauenfeld, Switzerland. He recognized the great significance of the diencephalon or mid-brain for the functions of the unconscious nervous system and, with it, the emotional. He was awarded the Nobel Prize in 1949 for his important medical discoveries.

The fact that by no means all mental diseases could be related to pathological-anatomical changes in the brain, led to the distinction between 'endogenic' and 'symptomatic' mental diseases. The man who brought methodical order into the confusion still reigning among the psychoses was a psychiatrist, Emil Kraepelin, who was born in 1855 in Neustrelitz and who can be regarded as the true founder of clinical psychiatry. He was director of the psychiatric clinics attached to the universities of Heidelberg and Munich and it was in Munich that he died in 1926.

While pathological processes have to this day only rarely been observed in the brain in endogenic psychoses, they regularly accompany symptomatic psychoses. One such symptomatic psychosis in which the connection between the physical and the mental is especially clear is dementia paralytica, a mental disease which, in 1857, Willers Jessen, a psychiatrist from Kiel, recognized as a condition following syphilis. Another German pioneer in skin and venereal diseases – who died much too prematurely – was Felix von Baerensprung, whose position in medical history can be compared with that of the Austrian pioneer of dermatology and syphilology, Ferdinand von Hebra (see page 257) who was six years his senior. A tragic fate ordained that von Baerensprung, who was born in 1822, the son of the chief burgomaster of Berlin, himself contracted dementa paralytica. Irregular bouts of derangement, excitement and hallucinations made it necessary for him to be admitted into the Hornheim Hospital near Kiel. On 26 August 1864 when he was only forty-two years old he took his own life; not far from the Kiel Palace he threw himself into the sea.

A great number of intellectually distinguished men were carried off by this terrible, paralytic disease during the second half of the nineteenth and the first years of the twentieth century. To mention only a few of them – Hugo Wolf, the composer; the 'saviour of mothers', Ignaz Philipp Semmelweis (see page 260); the writer, Guy de Maupassant; the philosopher, Friedrich Nietzsehe; the poet, Nikolaus Lenau; and others.

The long, drawn-out death in years of mental darkness and physical decay was terrible; but however hard the young science of psychiatry tried to help the wretched paralytics, all efforts proved unsuccessful. Among those who were not satisfied with the prevailing methods of treating mental illness was a young assistant doctor who was working at the psychiatric clinic of Vienna University in the 1880s. His name was Julius Wagner-Jaurreg and he had been born in 1857 in Wels, Upper Austria. The young twenty-five-year-old doctor was most depressed by the sad cases of young mothers who, during delivery or shortly afterwards, fell victim to acute attacks of derangement or delirium.

Wagner-Jaurreg spent many an hour pondering how best to help these unfortunate women. Whatever he tried, however, proved unsuccessful until one day, chance gave him a clue. One of the women patients in his clinic, who was suffering from pregnancy psychosis, fell ill with a feverish attack of typhus and, as if by magic, the mental darkness vanished, although only temporarily. At first the young assistant doctor believed this was just a coincidence; but his attention was aroused when another, equally hopelessly deranged mother was completely cured as a result of surviving an attack of erysipelas of the head, accompanied by high fever.

The possibility that fever might possess healing power haunted Wagner-Jaurreg. He collected relevant case histories from both ancient and recent writings, assiduously continued his own observations and, in 1887, the thirty-year-old doctor published a scientific work on the favourable effect of fever on mental illness. In it he suggested artificially engendering a 'healing fever' by infecting hopeless cases with erysipelas or malaria.

His suggestion was ignored; but Wagner-Jaurreg did not falter. At first he worked with tuberculin in order to ameliorate various different mental diseases by means of the 'healing fever' but his successes proved modest. Therefore, he turned his attention to the well-outlined, symptomatic psychosis of dementia paralytica. During the years 1907, 1908 and 1909 he treated altogether eighty-six paralytics with tuberculin fever; and when, several years later, in 1915, he published a scientific report on the results of this treatment, it was demonstrated that of the eighty-six, twenty-one were still alive and a third of these were following their former professions. This was certainly not an overwhelming result; but considering that the paralysis would otherwise have resulted in death after a few years in practically all cases, it was nevertheless a success deserving some respect. But still no one took the slightest notice.

During the First World War a soldier from the Balkan front came into Wagner-Jaurreg's clinic with malaria. Fate itself had offered the indefatigable research scientist a possibility of putting into practice his old plan of treatment for paralytics by artificial infection with malaria. Wagner-Jaurreg did not hesitate. On 14 June 1917 he hazarded the important step and injected malaria microbes into the bloodstream of two mortally ill paralytics. During the following eight weeks a further seven otherwise hopeless cases of paralysis were also artificially infected with malarial fever, so that Wagner-Jaurreg now had at his disposal nine cases.

Ten years later three of these nine 'incurable' cases were completely well and going out to work; a third of his patients had therefore been treated with success. Indefatigably, Wagner-Jaurreg carried on his work and discovered that the reason for the small proportion of cures was merely that the treatment had, in the other cases, been started too late. In fact, after starting the malaria-fever therapy at an earlier stage, he succeeded in improving the percentage of recoveries. Success was even more conspicuous if, at the same time as the artificial malaria infection, a course of Salvarsan was also carried out – just as if, as a result of the fever, the virus had become more easy to fight with chemo-therapeutic measures.

Thus Wagner-Jaurreg, in his time, created for medical science a weapon against paralysis, and for this feat he was awarded the Nobel Prize for Medicine in 1927. Wagner-Jaurreg died when he was eighty-three; and even though, in the meantime, this paralysis has become a rare disease and one which is today treated with antibiotics, Wagner-Jaurreg's name will never be forgotten by medical historians.

If the theory of the actual nervous diseases was still counted as belonging to the realms of 'internal medicine' until the second half of the last century, it was a German scientist who created a separate discipline, neurology. His name was Wilhelm Heinrich Erb and he was born in Heidelberg in 1840. The house in which he was born stands in Winweiler in the Palatinate. Even as a growing boy he was unusually hard-working, reliable and eager to learn. When he was seventeen he was admitted to the Heidelberg University. He passed the medical state examination in Munich and when he was twenty-two returned to Heidelberg as an assistant at the medical clinic in the university. Soon the young doctor began to perform experiments based on his own ideas; but he never felt as drawn to other faculties as he did to the discipline of nervous diseases.

His research into the electrical treatment of diseases, which was still in its infancy, produced such a wealth of valuable results that Erb was soon able to publish a *Handbook of Electrotherapy and Electrodiagnostics* which for the first time gave scientific status to this new branch of research. However the author did not rest on his laurels. Tirelessly, purposefully, driven on by relentless research activity, he reaped one fruit after another from the many-branching tree of neurology which he had himself planted. At a time when no one knew anything about hormones and vitamins, he discovered that, during the convulsive disease, tetanus, the excitability of the motor nerves is considerably heightened, and science has rewarded him for this knowledge by, to this day, describing this symptom as 'Erb's phenomenon'. Erb discovered the tendon reflex, knowledge of which is now a matter of course for every medical man; he made clear the connection between syphilis and the other great luetic disease, *Tabes dorsalis* (progressive locomotor ataxia), and recognized that the loss of pupil reflexes was an early symptom of this dreadful affliction. He was also the first to demonstrate that certain attacks of limping were caused by a deterioration of the leg arteries. In 1880 Wilhelm Erb was appointed director of the Neurological Clinic in the University of Leipzig; later, however, he felt impelled to return to his beloved Heidelberg where he worked as director of the medical clinic at the university from 1883 to 1907. No appointment, however, brilliant, could tempt him away from there.

He was granted in full measure all the honours which a successful scientist and researcher could receive; he became an honorary member of numerous medical societies, was made a privy councillor with the title 'excellency'; the Grand Duke of Baden awarded him the highest order in his power; an Erb commemorative medal was struck, to be awarded every two years to the writer of the best work on neurology; and the time during which he was active was called the 'Periclean era of neurology'.

In spite of all this, Wilhelm Erb remained unaffected and home-loving; he loved company, music and the beauties of his Palatinate homeland, the Black Forest and Switzerland. Notwithstanding the stupendous results of his research, Wilhelm Erb – who died in Heidelberg in 1921 at the age of eighty-one after leading a full, active life – was never a fanatic for work in the bad sense of the word. He was responsive to the joys of life and once gave his assistant, who was later to become the famous Hamburg nerve doctor, Max Nonne, the following piece of valuable advice: 'A life devoted only to work is not a full life; work hard and play hard!'

In spite of the progress made as a result of research on the healthy and disordered nervous system, ideas about the nature of diseases conditioned by nerves were still widely divergent. Towards the end of the last century, doctors in Vienna still believed in a purely physical cause for mental disease; in Paris, on the other hand, something of Mesmer's 'animal magnetism' still survived and here it was the prominent clinician at the Salpêtrière, Jean Martin Charcot (1825–1893) who made the observation that symptoms of hysteria could be produced by hypnosis.

This discovery, that physical conditions could be conjured up by mental conceptions, made a great impression on a man who was destined to create a whole new method of treatment for neuroses; Sigmund Freud. Born on 6 May 1856 in Freiburg, Moravia, he studied medicine from 1873 to 1881 and, with his colleague, Dr Joseph Breuer, began to take an interest in psychopathology and psychotherapy in 1883. Breuer and Freud had been able to cure patients suffering from hysteria by encouraging them to talk, and soon Freud was positive that hysteria was not brought about by a physical, organic defect, but as a result of inner conflicts of which the patient himself was unaware. This perception caused Freud to set himself the task of 'exploring the subconscious part of the individual psychic life'. The 'psycho-analysis' which developed from this, took the form of the patient telling the doctor, during the course of conversations, about earlier experiences which had been suppressed.

Freud's theory, however revolutionary its effect may have been, and however many disciples – especially in America – it may have had, suffered from one-sided, over-emphasis on the sexual. According to Freud, neuroses spring up wherever 'as a result of external or internal checks, the satisfaction of the erotic needs is denied in reality'. Against this thesis is the fact of medical experience that there are countless people who cannot satisfy their innermost, secret, erotic wishes, and consequently have to work them off mentally but, nevertheless, do not suffer from neuroses. Freud was forced to emigrate from Vienna to London when he was eighty-two where he died, on 23 September 1939 at the age of eighty-three.

337

Physiology and pathology of the brain and nervous system were further augmented by the electro-encephalograph invented by the German neurologist and psychiatrist, Hans Berger (1873–1941). This instrument, which, in the same way that the electro-cardiograph records the action currents of the heart, registers the electrical currents caused by brain activity.

An interesting relationship between the endogenic psychoses and individual types of body-structure was found by Ernst Kretschmer, a psychiatrist from Tübingen (1888–1964) who, in an extended series of examinations, was able to establish that schizophrenia favours people of slender build, whereas manic-depressive madness is more likely to occur in people who are more portly.

In spite of the fact that, in various ways, scientists were coming closer to unravelling the functions of the healthy and the diseased brain, the endogenic psychoses in particular remained and still remain shrouded in countless impenetrable mysteries. This is demonstrated by the uncertainty and frequent change in methods of treatment. Shock therapy with electric currents is a rigorous measure and anyone who has seen how patients are led to this treatment with its attendant insulin, cardiazol and other spasm-producing drugs, will not quite be able to avoid making an agonizing comparison with the violent methods used in the past. No less drastic seems the 'psycho-surgical' method of treatment, the frontal lobotomy or leukotomy, in which a special two-edged knife severs the connection between the frontal lobe and the rest of the brain. Although the initiator of this method, Antonio Moniz, was awarded the Nobel Prize for his discovery in 1949, his procedure, which was accompanied by a personality change and made people resemble automatons, has since been abandoned.

However, it now looks as if, through the young science of psycho-pharmacology, a change in the treatment of psychoses is on its way. After science had got to know the so-called 'hallucinogenic' substances, only minute doses of which can reproduce in completely healthy people confusingly exact symptoms of schizophrenia, psycho-pharmacologists set themselves to find substances which might counter the hallucinogenic substances created in the organism itself, perhaps as a result of metabolic lapses.

The first clear results of this endeavour are chlopromazin, as also the alkaloid, Reserpin, which is obtained from the root-coverings of the Indian plant *Rauwolfia serpentina* which was already being used thousands of years ago (see page 54). Because of their suppressive effect on psychotic conditions of excitement, both medicines now are part of the normal equipment of psychiatric clinics. After these welcome first results, a veritable flood of 'psycho-medicines' began to be manufactured – at first in America – and a great many people lapsed into the belief that they could not live without their 'tranquillizers'. The misuse of such psycho-medicines very quickly began to threaten public health because of the addictive dangers which constant haphazard usage brought with it.

Thus, the science of 'mental medicines' still leaves much to be desired. One thing, however, can be said for it: since psycho-pharmacology became one of the healing methods used by psychiatrists, the atmosphere in the mental hospitals has completely changed.

41

*Progress in surgery; Emil Theodor Kocher
in Bern. Harvey Cushing develops neuro-
surgery. Ferdinand Sauerbruch and his
difference of pressure procedure. The
discovery of cortisone. Hans Selye founds
the 'stress' theory of the 'adaptive diseases'.
Spare-parts surgery and the transplant of
organs. The first heart transplant.*

The green light for rapid ad-
vances in surgery was given when doctors had discovered how
to eliminate pain from operations; when the German surgeon,
Ernst von Bergmann, had improved upon Lister's antisepsis and
produced asepsis; when the Parisian surgeon, Jules Péan (1830–
1898) had invented the artery forceps – which, to this day, bear
his name – so that haemostasis (blood staunching) presented no
further problem; when the Viennese serologist, Karl Landsteiner,
at the beginning of this century, removed all danger from
blood-transfusions by his discovery of blood groups (see page
302) and, finally, when roentgenology, by making use of opaque
meal, had perfected the diagnosis of the internal cavities.

At the frontier, so to speak, of the new surgical era, stood the
distinguished Swiss operating surgeon, Emil Theodor Kocher
(1841–1917), who was director of the surgical clinic at the
University of Bern. Uniquely, Kocher had become a specialist
in the surgical removal of the goitres which were so prevalent in

his country. He was the first to recognize the true causes of the serious clinical picture accompanying a too radical removal of the thyroid gland or the removal (or damaging) of the parathyroid and in so doing he made a valuable contribution to the theory of internal secretions.

At this time, the United States energetically began to make contributions to the development of medicine, and American surgeons were in the news for the first time. One of these men, who deserves special mention, was Harvey Cushing. From 1905, he made considerable advances in the field of neuro-surgery. After finishing his training in American universities, Cushing – who was born in Cleveland, Ohio in 1869 – continued his studies both in London and with Kocher in Bern; he was always to remember his student years with special affection. 'In this lovely city,' he wrote, 'I experienced, at the turn of the century, a thoroughly enjoyable and productive period of my medical education at the Insel-spital and Hallerianum.' At the end of the First World War, Cushing was at the peak of his scientific fame. At the International Medical Congress, which took place in 1919, he said: 'Brain surgery only made rapid progress after the neurologists had begun to build up their own system of surgery.' When the International Day of Neurology was held in Bern, in 1931, he could report on the proud results of two thousand operations for tumour of the brain, with a comparatively low rate of mortality of 11.9 per cent. Cushing, who was famous for his extremely careful way of operating – which was described as a 'silk technique' – died in 1939; he, too, had enriched the theory of internal secretions by the discovery of a hormone disease, which was named after him and which was caused by a tumour on the adrenal cortex or the hypophyse.

A German surgeon, Ferdinand Sauerbruch (1875–1951) introduced a new era into the surgery of the pleural cavity. As a result of the differential pressure procedure which he invented, it became possible to open the thorax in a low-pressure chamber, without the lung collapsing and respiration ceasing. Even though, today, the differential pressure procedure has been replaced by endotracheal narcosis and artificial bronchial respiration, Sauerbruch will always be remembered as one of the most energetic promoters of surgery in medical history.

At that time, the lead in the development of medicine was transferred more and more clearly to the United States of America. Once again, it was an important and practical discovery which brought the theory of internal secretions into the foreground of medical interest. In 1948 – Germany was still cut off from all foreign, especially American, research as a result of the Second World War – Philip S. Hench, a doctor at the world-famous Mayo Clinic in Rochester, Minnesota, discovered that both pregnancy and jaundice generally exercised a favourable influence on chronic inflammatory rheumatism or 'arthrosis'.* During the course of his research, Hench became more and more convinced that arthrosis was not a germ-produced disease but came about as a result of biochemical disturbances in the body and that these disturbances could be favourably affected by chance changes of condition, such as, for example, pregnancy, jaundice, etc. From this assumption it was only a step to the conclusion that it must be the *same* substance in both pregnancy and jaundice which brought about the improvement.

It was soon conjectured that this substance must be one of the adrenal hormones. This was because other measures which stimulated the internally secreting functions of the adrenal glands as, for example, narcosis, surgical intervention, etc., could also produce a temporary relief in cases of arthrosis. Therefore Hench got in touch with Edward Calvin Kendall, a biochemist also working at the Mayo Foundation, who discovered the thyroid hormone (see page 314) and in September 1948 a young chemist in Kendall's laboratory called Sarrett succeeded in synthesizing a small amount of an entirely new active substance which was called cortisone. Thereby the foundation had been laid for the

* From *arthron* – the Greek for joint; chronic inflammation of the joint

creation of a whole new group of medical substances whose further development was to prove highly fruitful for medical science. In 1950 Philip S. Hench and Edward C. Kendall were awarded the Nobel Prize for this achievement.

The early excitement over cortisone was, it is true, somewhat dampened when it turned out that the improvement only lasted as long as the drug was being administered. The whole procedure threatened to fall into disrepute when, in 1955, American research scientists succeeded in dehydrating cortisone under the influence of micro-organisms. This resulted in the creation of cortisone derivatives which could be taken orally in tablet form and considerably extended the range of application. The 'classic' disease susceptible to cortisone treatment, chronic rheumatic endocarditis, has long stopped being the exclusive disease treated by the new preparations; they also act with considerable reliability on Addison's disease (a disease caused by the hypofunction of the thyroid), gout, asthma, hay fever and other conditions due to hypersensitivity; they are also used when extraordinary demands are placed on the body, such as the results of operations, accidents and the like, as well as in many other kinds of diseases.

Finally, the discovery of cortisone called up a whole new subjective concept of disease: the theory of stress, originated by the Austro-Canadian doctor, Hans Selye. Selye, who was born in Vienna in 1907, studied in Prague, Paris and Rome and, after his emigration to the New World, took over the directorship of the Institute for Experimental Medicine and Surgery at the University of Montreal in 1945. According to Selye, every time an extraordinary load or demand (stress) is imposed on an organism, an unspecific general 'syndrome* of being ill' sets in. The reactions caused by over-exertion can be of various kinds: infections, injuries, burning, poisoning, radiations, muscular over-exertions, psychological excitement, etc. After systematic research, Selye succeeded in explaining the effect caused by the defensive

* Group of symptoms

measures with which the organism opposes the 'stress'. What pointed the way was the fact that during the 'syndrome of being ill' the cortex of the adrenal gland is generally enlarged. When a stress, of no matter what kind, affects the organism, the pituitary gland or hypophysis pumps out a hormone which stimulates the adrenal gland to increased production of its active substance. Since the adrenal hormones such as cortisone exercise a far-reaching influence on the various functions of the organs, for example by regulating the sugar and mineral supply, they can also develop a lasting effect on symptoms.

'Adaptive' diseases are brought about if the interplay of active substances, which Selye called 'adaptive hormones' is not functioning properly. The most common adaptive diseases are complaints affecting the heart and circulation, such as high blood pressure, myocardial infarction; gastric ulcers, and skin diseases such as psoriasis, and allergic conditions or diseases of hypersensitivity. All these adaptive diseases are, therefore, according to Selye, not caused directly by a disease-bearing germ, but are brought about – according to the reaction of the individual human organism – by the fact that the adaptive hormones confronting the stress are in some way disturbed.

Hans Selye's theory of stress has already been found of practical use, for in severe, stress-causing, perilous conditions of shock or collapse, soluble compounds of cortisone are injected into the veins, by which means many lives are saved.

The most recent medical development is especially distinguished by the immense advances made in surgery, where the achievements at times seem almost miraculous. True, they would not have been possible if important preconditions for the success of modern operating techniques had not first been created; such as preparation before an operation, the refinement of the pain-killing processes and finally, also, the combating of shock. Medical technical science which is today also in the midst of a magnificent process of development, whose consequences it is not yet entirely possible to survey, has done one thing more: it has given to

344

medicine a number of revolutionary apparatuses, machines and instruments and, as a result, opened up realms of surgery which, without such technical help, no surgeon would have ever dared to approach. Already, several American universities have professorships for biological/medical/technology; the further developments in this field cannot yet be foreseen.

Through the creation of the heart-lung machine, the most difficult heart operations, such as the artificial replacement of a heart-valve, have become possible; today thousands of people are walking around with artificial heart-valves made of Silastik, synthetic material that is not rejected by the living organism. Electrical pacemaker machines are set into the pleural cavity to govern the constant stimulation or regulation of the disturbed activity of the heart. A research scientist in Cleveland is even working at the construction of an artificial heart made entirely of plastic that is likely to be fully developed in several years' time. Artificial kidneys are already keeping alive people whose own kidneys have failed. True, this process still has one major disadvantage: the kidney patient must report at least once a week to a 'kidney centre' there his blood circulation is connected to the artificial kidney for a certain length of time and, through dialysis – the separation of chemical substances – the waste products can be filtered off outside the body. Hosever, biological medical/technology is already at work trying to construct handy small artificial kidneys which the patient can constantly carry around in his pocket. By 1968 this work had proceeded so far that an 'artificial kidney for the sitting room' was already in existence. This kidney-in-the-home is of a fairly handy format, weighs 4.6 kg., costs about £3,000 and can be looked after by the relatives of the kidney patient without any difficulty.

Beside this 'spare-parts' medicine, however, there is also transplant surgery, which makes use either of the patient's own, or another person's organs, in a totally amazing development. In

Canada a surgical treatment has recently been developed for angina pectoris, in which the coronary vessels of the heart have deteriorated or become convulsed. In this, a part of the 'net' which hangs like a curtain in front of the abdominal viscera, and is well supplied with blood-vessels, is transplanted on to the heart and tied to the aorta; the blood-vessels in the 'net' then grow into the heart muscle, giving it a stronger supply of blood and oxygen. Blood-vessels which have degenerated can be replaced by transplants; and so, just as there are blood banks for blood-transfusions, there are also banks for arteries and other organs as well.

Transplant surgery, which makes use of the super-cooled 'foreign' organs of people who have died in accidents, would probably have advanced much further if it were not for one obstacle which keeps confronting it: the defence mechanism of the organism against 'foreign' albumen, which is an indication that the blood groups discovered by Karl Landsteiner (see page 301) are apparently only a small part of the biological differences separating one individual from another. However, even this 'immunity' barrier will be overcome one day – perhaps very soon, for already substances to curb the transplant rejection are known. Already doctors have dared to make kidney and liver, pancreas and lung transplants even though the survival time of the operated patients is as yet still short.

At the end of 1967, Professor Christian Barnard, a surgeon in Cape Town, South Africa, even succeeded in transplanting the heart of an accident casualty into a patient whose own heart was on the point of failing. In 1968 other heart transplants were undertaken with varying success in the U.S.A., Japan and in Europe – for the first time in Paris, London and elsewhere.

Once the 'immunity barrier' is conquered and the rejection reaction arrested, a whole new era of medicine will dawn. For the necessity of having replacement organs constantly available will have the grim consequence of causing a radical revolution in conceptions held hitherto regarding the untouchable nature of the dead. These are by no means futuristic fantasies. It is no exaggeration to say that, in this respect, medical science is already in the middle of the revolution.

42

*Medicine of the future. The medical
computer. The 'electronic nurse'. Geriatrics
the urgent concern of present and future
medicine. The regression of infectious
diseases and increase of the degenerative
diseases. The art of the doctor is, according
to Hippocrates, 'of all the arts the most
distinguished'.*

If the most recent developments
in surgery are already pointing clearly into the future, the same
applies even more strongly to the most modern innovation in the
history of medicine – the use of electronics in the service of
healing. The medical computer, still a rarity in the Old World,
has already been fully developed in America. At the present time,
in the Mayo Clinic mentioned earlier, the case histories of the
two hundred thousand patients who are examined there annually
are already being electronically assessed. Medical robots are constructed by brilliant scientists in all medical specialist faculties,
who feed into the medical computers all their wealth of medical
knowledge broken down into the smallest detail. This involves
such a vast amount of data – there are forty thousand different
diseases – that no doctor in the world could keep all their symptoms in his head. The computer, however, stores them all up.
While he is still in the waiting room, the patient is handed a pile
of punched cards containing all the questions which a doctor

normally puts to his patient. He must answer each question plainly with a 'yes', 'no' or 'not known'; then the cards are handed over to the computer. The computer indicates with lightning speed what disease the given symptoms indicate, suggests a treatment, diet, etc.

The accuracy of diagnosis is said to be at least 95 per cent; and, since this procedure is especially suitable for mass examinations, as a preventive measure, the inventors of the medical computer are convinced that 'the electronic computer can give more benefits to mankind than has any other invention before it.'

The old-fashioned doctor, who may fear that this 'medical robot' will destroy the personal contact, the human relationship between doctor and patient, is told: 'Only in the computer age will it again be possible for a doctor to give his intensive personal attention to a patient, for then computers will free him from all the routine medical work.'

It is true that in one field of medical science – nursing – Europe already makes use of electronic procedures; the impetus for this has obviously come from the ever more pressing shortage of staff. More and more, in cases of serious illness or after operations, are big hospitals transferring an accurate, uninterrupted watch over the most important functions of life to an automatic centre of surveillance. Primarily, it constantly checks the conditions vital to life, i.e. blood pressure, pulse, rate of respiration, temperature, etc. The electronic nurse is by no means intended to replace the real nurse; it is only intended to take some of the work off the nursing personnel. Through the electronic, central, automatic control, which, when danger threatens, at once sends out visual and audible signals, the duty sister has constant control over the condition of the seriously ill patients in her charge.

Of medical development, too, it is possible to say 'the future has already begun.' A distinguished medical journal, having questioned hospital directors, made the following prediction of what hospitals will be like in a hundred years' time: heart, liver and kidney transplants will be everyday affairs; the patients will be put to sleep by electrical hypnosis, and eat deep-frozen food which can be heated in minutes. The respiration, pulse and blood pressure of every patient will be reported continuously to a central station – as a matter of course, rather than as a speciality. It will also be an everyday affair for medical computers to make diagnoses with 95 per cent accuracy and to suggest courses of therapy. Specialists from all over the world will take part in the treatment by means of long-distance television. The hospital itself will be a skyscraper with a helicopter parking area.

In view of the great advances which medicine has made, and which caused a well-known clinician to say that the medical sciences have made more progress in the last eighty years than during the rest of the many thousands of years of its evolution, the question poses itself as to whether, as a result of this mighty upswing, the number of diseases and patients has become any smaller.

This question must certainly be answered with considerable caution. That man's expectation of life has literally doubled in the last hundred years is due, among many other things, to medical progress, hygiene, dietetics, etc. Since, however, as a result there are more and more old people, it follows that the number of geriatric diseases is steadily on the increase. According to considered judgement, this increase will continue until 1980. It has, however, already had the effect of making geriatricians of more than half of all hospital doctors and specialists. A well-known clinician recently predicted that geriatrics would, in the foreseeable future, claim more interest than pediatrics.

Already, 35 percent of all bedridden patients in hospitals belong to the age group of sixty years and over. After the age of seventy there are almost no single diseases; in more than three-quarters of the cases, three, four or more diagnoses must be made simultaneously, for it is frequently a case of combined diseases which stand in close relationship to each other. The medicine of the future will, therefore, have to take an even greater interest

in the science of geriatrics and its treatment; and this is necessary
– quite apart from the question of the ethics involved – because of
the socio-political considerations, to ensure that the healthy
younger working population is not overburdened with high main-
tenance costs.

Modern geriatrics have already achieved a great deal. Beside
the polyvalent preparations made of ferments, hormones, vitamins
and minerals, there is a number of recently originated, delicate
geriatric operations – as, for example, the prevention of stroke by
an operation to remove the narrowing, or closing-up, of the
carotid which is the cause in almost a third of the cases of stroke;
or the treatment of senile gangrene, for which there was once
only one treatment – 'high' amputation – by replacing the imper-
meable leg artery with a transplant taken from an artery bank.
Even senile deafness has up to a point become treatable. Apart
from the electro-accoustic hearing-aids which are constantly being improved, there are already minute otological* operations
which can either make mobile again the auditory ossicles which
had become rigid, or substitute a new fenestra for the one that
has become closed between the middle and the inner ear.

On the other hand, geriatrics are still fairly powerless when
confronted by another trial which attacks old age – arthrosis. Every
day experience goes to show that damage to the joints becomes
worse with increasing age and, therefore, the doctor encounters
chronic joint conditions more and more frequently among his
patients as the average age goes up. When American research
discovered cortisone (see page 343), it was hoped that at last an
effective remedy against arthrosis had been found. However, as
already mentioned, events were soon to show that it could only
achieve relief from the pain, but not a cure of the arthrotic
condition.

However, if there can be no question of an actual retreat of
illness, the reason for this is not that specific geriatric diseases
are on the increase, but because – while the infectious diseases

* Pertaining to the ear

were controlled as a result of the discovery of sulphonamide and penicillin, and infant mortality reduced by preventive inoculation and the improvement of general hygiene – a number of degenerative diseases went on gaining ground. Among these are, beside the arthroses, chiefly those which have grown out of arteriosclerotic conditions, including those affecting the heart or circulatory system – which are ever on the increase; also subconscious neuroses, gastric ulcers, obesity, slipped or damaged discs, and last but by no means least in this sad list, the malignant growths. Diabetes must also be mentioned in this connection; its slow but steady rate of increase shows that although progress in medical knowledge may help the individual patient, the total number of sufferers continues to increase.

Today, the chief concern of medicine is for those groups of diseases which are the leaders of the statistical causes of death: the heart-circulatory diseases and cancer. Among the circulatory conditions, arteriosclerosis holds pride of place in the clinician's and pathologist's interest; for almost all serious conditions of illness which come under this heading stem, in the last resort, from sclerotically degenerated blood-vessels: myocardial infarction the manifold types of disturbances to the circulation, the stroke and many other dangerous conditions. In spite of all intensive research, no clear certainty about the causes of vein calcination had been reached. Prominent experts on arteriosclerosis are of the opinion that an immoderate consumption of fat is the chief cause of degenerating arteries, and the conditions resulting from this. Other opinions blame the increasing use of manufactured sugar for heightening the disposition towards arteriosclerosis; especially significant, however, is said to be the coincidence of immoderate fat consumption with extremely high sugar intake as is often the case in the modern diet of so many people in the prosperous countries.

However, most recent research proves that a bad diet is without any doubt not the only cause of degenerating arteries. Overweight, blood pressure, chain-smoking of cigarettes, infections such as chronic tonsilitis, too little exercise and mental worries are additional causes and, with all of them, the still unknown great mystery called 'constitution' plays an important role. Since an effective treatment for arteriosclerosis, once it has set in, does not yet exist, modern prophylactic (preventative) medicine – which is still in course of development – has an especially responsible task to perform. Occupying second place among the statistical causes of death today are malignant growths – and it is one of the most tragic phenomena in the sphere of modern medicine that in spite of the most immense efforts which have been made in all civilized countries, nobody has yet succeeded in dealing with this scourge called cancer. Radiation and the knife are the only remedies – although all too often doubtful and merely temporary – which are employed and which, in any case, can only be used locally, and cannot stop the cancer as such. The experiments at present being intensively performed on cancer, using chemotherapy, have still not led to any satisfactory results.

The reasons for this are illuminating: the cancer growth consists of cells which are in a state of extraordinarily swift division. Therefore it is a question of finding chemical substances which can especially attack the rapidly increasing cells. Such substances have, in fact, already been synthesized, but now comes the reverse side of the coin: the healthy person also has at his disposal tissues with cells which are in a rapid process of division – for example, the blood-forming organs (the bone marrow produces about a billion red corpuscles daily). Therefore the 'cytostatics' (substances hindering cell multiplication) have the dangerous by-effect of damaging the blood-forming apparutus, and this fact prevents them from being more widely used at the present time.

The general practitioner is quite often told that modern medicine must really be considered incompetent, since it has still not been able to find a cure for cancer. Is that fair? There is doubtless a spark of truth in the statement, for if only a fraction of the countless milliards which are spent in building atom bombs and space ships were spent on cancer research, then medical science

353

would be much further on in the battle against one of the worst scourges of mankind. And should not man, before reaching for foreign stars, set all in order on his own planet?

Even though the chemotherapy of malignant growths is still only in its infancy – its initiator, Gerhard Domagk (see page 320) promised the author of this book speedy, decisive successes – we can expect that the solution to the cancer problem will one day be found in this sector. In the meantime a physicist in Dresden, Professor Manfred von Ardenne, by his 'overheating therapy' is trying to find a way to make the life of a cancer patient bearable. In the capital of Saxony Professor von Ardenne runs a cancer research institute with a staff of three hundred, and his procedure is based on the fact that the cancer cell is slightly more sensitive to heat than the normal body cell. The announcement Professor von Ardenne made about the results of his method at the International Medical Day 1967 in Stockholm sounded most promising.

However, notwithstanding such partial results, there are still a number of unfulfilled dreams in medicine. No certain remedies have yet been found for either heart and circulatory complaints or for malignant growths; the immunity barrier, which opposes the transplant of 'foreign' organs, has so far not been entirely overcome. There is as little that can be done to combat one of the most common nervous diseases, multiple sclerosis, as there is for leukaemia. Even such everyday diseases as arthrosis, paradentosis or subconscious neuroses can, at best, be eased, not cured; the endogenic psychoses remain shrouded in impenetrable darkness both as regards their cause and as regards a practical way of curing them.

It is hard to escape the impression that many of the afflictions which, particularly in modern times, seem to have been growing alarmingly more prevalent, are positively favoured in establishment and progress by our super-civilization. Therefore, apart from concentrating on the prevention of disease, the most urgent task confronting medical science, both at present and in the future, should be the application of a counterbalance to the increasingly unnatural mode of life to which modern man is condemned in this technological age, and to preserve him from those influences which could damage his inheritance . . .

The purpose of this book was to show the development of medical science, sweeping on from ancient prehistoric times through the millennia like a broad river in constant movement, sometimes slow, sometimes, when outstanding personalities hastened its course, racing along. The latter trend was first apparent when, with Hippocrates, the history of medicine emerged into the light from the preceding darkness. Even though we may now know that the evolution of medicine by no means started with that ancient Greek – but, as described in the first chapters of this book, had already, in the days of the ancient civilizations of the Mediterranean, the Far East and Pre-Columbian America – made considerable strides towards a rational way of thinking and healing – in one respect the teachings of the 'father of medicine' have to this day remained an unqualified example to medical practice. This concerns the duty to follow medical ethics and also – no matter how high the value placed on individual research – not to lose sight of the total picture, in the conviction that it is nature which heals, the doctor's work only being undertaken in nature's service. So long as there are doctors in the civilized world, Hippocrates' words will remain true for them: 'The physician's art consists of three things: disease, patient and doctor. The doctor is the servant of the art, and the highest duty of the art of healing is to cure the patient. The art of healing is the most distinguished of all the arts.'

Index

Abel, Dr, 315
About Ancient Medicine, Hippocrates', 78
Ackerknecht, Erwin H., 80, 98, 214, 265
Acupuncture, in China, 46–7
Adrenalin, 314
Aesculapius, 25, 70–71
  ridiculed by Aristophanes, 72
Agrippa, Cornelius, 164
Akkadians, the, 21, 22
Al Rhazi, 109–10, 144
  his *El Hawl*, 110
Alcmaeon, Greek doctor, 69, 70, 75
Alexander the Great, 53, 69, 84, 86
Alexandria,
  decline of medicine in, 91
  founding and development, 87–8
  Galen in, 94
  taken by Arabs, 108
Allopathy, 253
Althoff, Friedrich, 306
American cultures, early, 58–9
Anaesthetics, 261, 262–4
  early, 263
Anatomy, 261, 262–4
  Aristotle's work, 85–6
  Bichat's work, 233–5
  developed in Alexandria, 87

Diocles' work, 82–3
  frowned on in Middle Ages, 116, 117
  Galen's work, 95
  Rokitansky's work, 255–6
  Sylvius's work, 189
  Vesalius' work, 141–5 *passim*
Andernach, Winter von, 144
Andromachus of Crete, 125
Antibiotics, 325
Antisepsis, 267–8
Arabic culture,
  absorbs Greek medicine, 108–9
  Arab doctors, 109–10
  development of Arab medicine, 109
  spread of Islam, 107–8
Ardenne, Prof. Manfred von, 354
Aristides, on Hippocrates, 74
Aristophanes, 72
Aristotle, 70, 83, 84, 86, 88, 97, 98
  errors, 85, 86, 173
  teaching, 84–5, 186
Arnold of Villanova, 115–16
Arthritis, primeval, 17–18
Ascheim, Dr, 315
Asclepiades of Cos, 75
Asclepiades of Prus, 91
Asepsis, 269
Assyrians, the, 22, 29

quarantines introduced, 126
Blood,
blood groups discovered,
301–2
blood vessels discovered, 178,
179–80, 181
circulation discovered in
China, 42
circulation discovered in
Europe, 168–9, 171–3
Boccaccio, Giovanni, 124
Body temperature, 186–7
Boerhaave, Herman, 194–6,
205, 206
Boniface VIII, Pope, 116
*Book on the Number Seven,
The*, 78
Bordeu, Theophile, 217
Borelli, Giovanni Alfonso, 186–
7
his *De Motu Animalum*, 187
Botany, and medicine, 155,
243–6
Bower, Colonel, 53
Brauell, Dr Friedrich, 286
Bretonneau, Pierre, 240
Breuer, Dr Joseph, 337
Broussais, François Joseph
Victor, 239–40
Brown-Séquard, Charles, 312–
13
Brunner, Johann Conrad, 182
Butenandt, Adolf, 315

Caesar, Julius, 91, 101
Caius, John, 150–51
Calvin, John, 167–8, 169, 170
victims of, 168

Cancer, 353
Carbolic acid, 268
Cathars, the, 157, 158
Cave of *Les Trois Frères*, 15–16,
18
Cells, human,
discovery of, 203–4
nucleus discovered, 243
work on, 243–4, 235–6
Ceram, C. W., 37
Chain, Dr Ernst Boris, 324
receives Nobel Prize, 325
Champollion, Jean-François, 37
Charana, Indian doctor, 53
Charcot, Jean Martin, 337
Charles I, King of England, 175
Charles II, King of England,
191
Charles V, Emperor, 143, 145,
146, 147
Charles VIII, King of France,
134, 135
Charles IX, King of France, 152
Chemotherapy,
founding of 303ff
of malignant growths, 354
Children's Crusades, 130–1
Chinese culture,
acupuncture, 46–7
anaesthetics, 263
ancient, 41–3
Chou dynasty, 43, 44, 45
doctors' examinations, 44
Han dynasty, 45–6
Manchu dynasty, 49
medical records, 43, 44
Moxa treatment, 47
pharmacopoeia, 48–9

Hammurabi, King of Babylon, 23
Harrington, Dr, 315, 317
Harvey, William, 146, 169, 176
  discovers circulation of blood, 171–3
  further studies, 174–5
  his *De Generatione Animalum*, 175
Head, Sir Henry, 46
Heart, the, 345
  transplants, 346
Hebra, Franz, 257, 259, 260
Helmholtz, Hermann, 272, 277-8
  his *Handbook of Physiological Optics*, 278
  his *Theory of Sound Perception*, 278
Hench, Philip S., 315, 342
  receives Nobel Prize, 343
Henle, Jacob, 272
  his *About the Miasmas and Contagions* etc., 261
Henri de Mondeville, 121
Henry II, King of France, 152
Henry VIII, King of England, 150, 151
Heraclides of Tarent, 90–91
Heresy, 158
  Church's attack on, 159
Herodotus,
  on Babylonian medicine, 30
  on Egyptian medicine, 36
Herophilus of Chalcedon, 88–9
  his *Anatomics*, 88
Hess, A. F., 311
Hess, Walter Rudolf, 332

receives Nobel Prize, 332
Hildegard von Bingen, 105
Hippocrates, 53, 69, 72, 73–4, 84, 96, 97, 98, 172, 190
  code, 75–6
  forms of treatment, 79–81
  on dietetics, 78
  qualities and philosophy, 74–7, 79, 81
  writings, 75
History of Living Creatures (Historia Animalum), Aristotle's, 84
Hittorf, Dr,
  discovers cathode ray, 300
Hodgkin, Thomas, 241
Hoernle, Dr, 54
Holbeins, the, 141
Holtz, Dr, 315
Holy Ghost, Order of the, 120
Homeopathy, 252–3
Homer, 67, 122
Hooke, Robert, 243
Hormones, 314, 315, 316, 317
Hospitallers, the (Order of the Hospital of St John), 120, 121
Huang-Ti, Emperor of China, 42
  his *Nei-ching*, 42, 44, 172
Hübotter, Franz, 43
Huneke, Dr Ferdinand, 46
Hunter, John, 208–9

Imhotep, Egyptian doctor and god, 33–4
Immunology,
  early work, 290–93

Spontaneous generation refuted, 216
Stanley, W. M., 328
Starling, Dr, 314
Stethoscope, 236
  invented, 237–8
Stolz, Friedrich, 314
Sulphonamides, 320–21, 325
Sumerian culture, 20, 21–2, 23
Sun Yat-Sen, 49
Surgery,
  advances in France, 207
  advances in last 100 years, 340–47
  anaesthetics, 262–4
  banned by Synod of Tours, 117
  hospital gangrene, 264–5
  Hunter's work, 208–9
  scientific basis established, 150–54
  transplant, 345–7
Susa, 23
Susruta, Indian doctor, 53, 54
Sweating sickness, English, 128, 151, 164
Sydenham, Thomas, 190
  military career, 191
  pioneers specific pathology, 192–3, 194
Sylvius (Franz de Boe), 189
Syphilis, 28, 150
  brought to Old World from New, 134–5
  Ehrlich's work on, 306–7
  origin of name, 135

Takamine, of Japan, 314

Templars, the (Order of the Knights of the Temple), 120, 127
Tetanus, 291, 293
Teutonic Knights, Order of the, 120
Theiler, Max, 329
  receives Nobel Prize, 329
Thermometer, clinical, 187
  invention of, 186
Thomas Aquinas, St, 119, 159
Thompson, R. Campbell, 22, 25
Tiberius, Emperor, 102
Tiedemann, Friedrich, 217–19
Titian, 127, 141, 144
Trachoma, in Ancient Egypt, 35
Trojan War, 67–8
  plague during, 122
Trousseau, Armand, 240
Tuberculosis, Koch's work on, 286, 289
Tutankhamen, Pharaoh, 35

Uhlenhut, Paul, 306, 307
Universal Surgery, A, Ambroise Paré's, 152
Universities,
  founding of the European, 114–15
  medieval medicine taught by priests, 115
Ur,
  King's burial chamber, 28
  medical records from, 20

Vaghbata, Indian doctor, 53